VIRTUAL CHILD

VIRTUAL CHILD

THE TERRIFYING TRUTH ABOUT
WHAT TECHNOLOGY IS DOING TO CHILDREN

BY CRIS ROWAN, BSCOT, BSCBI, SIPT

Sunshine Coast Occupational Therapy Inc.

Sunshine Coast Occupational Therapy Inc.
6840 Seaview Rd.
Sechelt, BC Canada V0N3A4

The Library of Congress has cataloged the soft cover edition as follows:

Rowan, Cris

Virtual Child: The terrifying truth about what technology is doing to children

Includes research references and index.

It is not the intention of the author to provide specific medical advice. The contents of this book are intended as useful information and are not a substitute for medical advice, diagnosis or treatment of any physical, mental, social or academic disorder. For advice, diagnosis or treatment of specific disorder in any of the aforementioned areas, readers should consult their own qualified medical or education expert. The author and publisher are not liable for any damages or negative consequences from any treatment, action, application or preparation undertaken by any person as a result of reading the information in this book. References are provided for information purposes only and do not constitute endorsement of any research, websites or other sources. Readers should be aware that the websites listed in this book may change.

ISBN – 13: 978-1453719527

Children are the future of our planet.
Through modern technology, we have unconsciously created a virtual reality for our children to call home, a reality devoid of connection and human interaction.

Televisions, video games and the internet are now the teachers of our children, not parents. The result has been an alarming increase in attachment and developmental disorders.

Now is the time to plant the seed for children to learn in a new and conscious way. Teaching children to bring awareness to themselves, so they know who they are, creates a strong healthy foundation for learning.

Using their energy in positive productive ways, children learn to create balance and wholeness of body, mind and spirit.

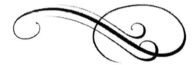

This book is dedicated to children everywhere, who want to find their spirit and soar.

Contents

Foreword - Our Ship Has Set Sail

Words of Wisdom from an Ancient Philosopher

Could I climb to the highest place in Athens, I would lift my voice and proclaim:
"Fellow citizens, why do ye turn and scrape every stone to gather wealth, and take so little
care of your children, to whom one day you will relinquish it all?"

Socrates

I was raised very well. I grew up spending a lot of time outside, especially in my younger years. From the stormy shores of the Queen Charlotte Islands to the calm waters of Desolation sound, from my father's sailboat, to my mother's kayaks, to my grandparents' cabin, I grew up knowing what it was like to be in nature. I got to run through the woods, hike up mountains, and explore the ocean depths with a scuba tank on my back.

As I neared the end of high school the world seemed too big for me and I wasn't sure what I wanted to do. When the Army recruiters came to our school I was intrigued. Eventually, I was sold; dazzled by the flashy uniforms and promises of adventure, I decided to sign up. I attended university at the Royal Military College of Canada in Kingston, Ontario. The college was and still is located on a windy little peninsula on the shores of Lake Ontario.

While at the College I learned to do a wonderful number of things from playing ice hockey, to studying Shakespeare, to running across the frozen lake into town without getting caught. Kingston was a great town with lots of great little pubs and clubs and a fair amount of social activity. To escape the stresses of school, my friends and I would often gather at a small stream a short distance away from the campus grounds, a place we eventually would come to call "The Nook." We gathered here to relax, connect, and pontificate about the nuances of existence. It was a calming place with the sound of running water always casting a magical feel about it.

College was not all idealistic stories and time well spent, however. I also played my fair share of video games. I wasted countless hours blasting away at aliens in *Halo* or waging space battles in *Starcraft*. I never really ever thought of the games as bad or a waste of time, but there were many nights blown away by computer pixels. I even became borderline antisocial at times.

Since graduating from college and becoming a Naval Officer, I kind of quit playing video games. I'll still indulge on occasion with friends, but any time I play on my own I usually feel kind of sucked in, like I could be out doing something more productive, or meaningful. This disinterest in video games probably, in part, had something to do with the year and a half I spent rooming with a guy after college. "Joe" liked his video games and television a lot. I progressively watched him form a well defined groove in the couch from where he sat and gamed and watched football. Joe used to be a really fun guy; he taught me how to play golf and the times we went out and partied together were fun, but these times were slowly overtaken by him being glued to the couch. Eventually, I simply could not be in a house where the TV was always on. So I moved out.

There's nothing wrong with TV and video games, as long as they are kept within balance. The problem I see these days for kids and people in general is an over reliance on technology. Cell phones and iPods annoy me to no end, because they make it so hard just to have a simple conversation with someone. To me, someone wearing iPod headphones or texting on their phone pretty much says "don't talk to me; I'm busy." Now, even Facebook, or "Face Crack" as some of my friends call it, is taking the place of people calling one another and simply talking on the phone with them. A girl recently told me she had some of her "friends" send her a wedding invitation on Facebook! Unbelievable!

What I've also found astounding from reading Mom's book *Virtual Child*, is the sheer amount of technology that parents and teachers are subjecting their kids to, and the possibly very damaging effects that this technology may have on our children. Kids need to be raised and loved by humans, not technology. Parents need to connect with their kids, just like people need to connect with people. We live in a social, physical world, one that needs to be explored, traveled, and, above all, enjoyed. People were never evolutionarily designed to sit in front of a TV and avoid all social contact. Sure it's fun to blast aliens from time to time and engage in fantasy, but doing it all the time will render us slaves to technology, just like in the *Matrix* movies, simply *plugged in*, and waiting to be woken up.

As humans, we must remember that we are in control of our own lives. One of my greatest teachers at college explained to us how in the 18th and 19th centuries, when the modern day novel was literally being *invented*, humans, philosophers, and writers believed that humanity was like a ship, a great arc that spanned time and space. This ship was full of humankind's ideas, feelings, and memories. This ship's course, this ship's *rudder* was the direction that humanity was going. These people believed that they could control humanity's values and, in the end, where the world was headed. They were truly great philosophers and intellectuals.

In present day, I often get the feeling like humanity isn't quite envisioning the direction it is headed. The ice caps are melting, the tar sands tailing ponds are still draining into the Athabaskan River and we keep driving. We're too busy to take care of our kids so we put them in front of the TV. We're pinching every penny so we buy chicken breasts that come from a bird that lives in a one square foot box and is injected with growth hormones every day. The western world is at risk of becoming a slave to the "mill run" life it has created for itself. Our ship has set sail, but do the people on board have any idea where it is headed?

In a way, technology and mass production have become a super powered engine that is driving our ship faster than we can steer it. It has connected the world through the internet and mobile communications; yet, it has somehow disconnected us as well. Are three people sitting together, one playing with their iPod, one texting and the other just sitting there, really together, or are they all just waiting for something to happen?

Social connection is the means through which humans share ideas, feelings, and touch. It is the warmth through which we survive as a species. If our generation and those that come to follow us are to survive in our increasingly challenging and physical world, we must remain connected to one another, to ourselves, and to our planet. This means that we can't let ourselves be constantly plugged into a bright display screen. This means we must venture out more often and see what the fresh air of the day has to offer. This means we must teach and raise our kids right, with a balanced approach to technology. This means we must read this book, and learn how.

Thanks Mom!
Matt Taccogna, Navy Lieutenant and Author's Son
Victoria, British Columbia
28 October, 2010

Prologue - Connection to Technology Is Disconnecting Children

On October 21st, 2008, following an argument with his Dad over the confiscation of his X-box 360, a 15 year old boy from Barrie Ontario named Brandon Crisp steered his bike away from home. Three weeks later Brandon's body was found 6 kilometers from his home under a tree. Autopsy reports indicate Brandon died of chest injuries sustained in a fall. Why did Brandon ride so far away from home in sub-zero weather and climb a tree?

Globe and Mail, October 22, 2008.

It is a widely held belief by society that technologies such as television, internet, video games and cell phones are harmless, and children with dependencies can just be "unplugged" whenever adults want, without long term or devastating consequences. It is now estimated that up to 10% of elementary children are addicted to video games, with some as young as two years of age. Underlying these addictions is a pervasive and endemic ailment of 21st century society – the preference of a device over human beings. As children are connecting more and more to technology, they are disconnecting from humanity. Children are spending long hours immersed in dark and lonely virtual worlds, disconnecting not only from themselves, but also from their family, friends, classmates and even their pets. While the family dog is ignored and chained in the back yard, children raise virtual avatar pets on *Second Life*. Streets and parks are empty and quiet now, as children move deeper and deeper into their virtual worlds.

This "disconnection" by children isn't just from themselves and others. They now fear nature and being in the Great Outdoors. Scouts Canada numbers are now half what they were only a decade ago. The worst disconnection though, one that will change the path of humanity forever is a disconnection of children from their spirit. No longer do we hear the joys of laughter as children play games outside. Nor do we see the spark in children's eyes as they learn to ride their bike, or build imaginary cities in the dirt and people out of sticks and leaves. Everyone is obsessed with escaping from their present stressed existence, but to where, and why?

In the history of humankind, there has never been such rapid change to systems and structures used that govern our lives. The very fabric we used to build our home, school, work, and community systems is unraveling, leaving humans struggling to adapt. The intrusion of technology into human lives has hit us so fast and with such force, that there has been little time to plan how to accommodate the profound change technology has made to our lives. Teachers have now quit teaching printing, and reading is taught on-screen. As books become a thing of the past, curriculum is administered on "XOs" or "TeacherMates". Can we remove the human *flesh and blood* teacher and expect children to actually learn and achieve literacy with an electronic device? Maybe in the new age world, printing, reading and numerical literacy are just a thing of the past, and won't be necessary for our children's future. We simply do not know.

Can we replace human parents as primary attachment figures with a device as well? As parents become more and more attached to their own various forms of technology, they are detaching from their children. Whether at home, school or in the community, children are encouraged to immerse themselves in gadgets, but at what cost to their physical, mental, social and academic success? Biologically speaking, can the human species detach from each other and attach to devices, and survive?

While the answers to many of these questions are largely speculative, I don't believe that our species is adapting to technology as well as we would like to think. In fact, technology overuse may have already surpassed the human capacity to adapt. Critical milestones for child sensory and motor development are not being met, and consequently attaining literacy has become problematic. In many ways, technology has already destroyed the fragile fabric that holds family and education systems together. As traditional family systems and structures devolve, isolated and lonely children form unhealthy attachments with technology. Educators in the school system are escalating their use of computers as tools for teaching children without evidence to support this initiative, nor sufficient research regarding long term outcomes. As limited education funding is diverted to technology, playgrounds – the epicenter for socialization and child development - fall into disrepair.

The new millennium has borne witness to rising incidence of child physical, mental, social, and academic disorders that the health and education systems are just beginning to detect, much less understand. One in three children exhibit health problems and/or learning difficulties, and one in six have been diagnosed with a mental illness, often accompanied by use of psychotropic medication. Exposure to an average of 7.5 hours per day of various forms of technology has resulted in a physically sedentary yet chaotically stressed existence for children.

The sustainability of our children's future is now in question. In the history of humankind, our children have never been sicker than they are right now. Technology may pose the largest threat ever to the health and well being of 21st century children, yet few people are willing to do something to counteract technology's pervasive presence in our children's lives. Developmentally delayed, learning disabled, obese, sleep deprived, mentally ill, isolated, aggressive, illiterate, and unable to pay attention, the new millennium child may be the first generation ever to not out live their parents.

In this book by a pediatric occupational therapist Cris Rowan, the disconnection of children from self, others, nature and spirit is profiled. The current status of child physical, mental, social and academic performance is revealed, and three critical milestones for achieving optimal child growth and success are reviewed. Research regarding the impact of technology overuse on child performance indicators is presented, and issues of concern for parents, health and education professionals regarding technology overuse by children are outlined. The future sustainability of children is analyzed. A variety of novel interventions and treatment approaches are recommended for private and public sectors to begin to manage balance between activities children need for growth and success with technology use.

Introduction - Why You Need To Read This Book

Over the past decade pediatric occupational therapists working in school-based settings have witnessed an astounding increase in incidence of referrals for young children (Davidson, 2010). Back in the 1990s as a school-based occupational therapist, I managed a small caseload servicing a moderate to severely disabled population with diagnoses such as cerebral palsy, autism, down's syndrome, spinal bifida, and brain injury. Now referrals consist of predominantly printing and reading delays, attention and learning difficulties, and significant behavior problems. This sudden influx of child referrals into understaffed and wholly unprepared education and health care systems, has caused considerable workload management stress. In order to provide assistance to these children, well-meaning educators and therapists have placed these children into diagnostic categories with profound and far reaching consequences. The past decade has truly borne witness to profound changes in children, and its now time to ask the question: "Why"?

About five years ago, I started to query the role of technology use by children as a plausible cause in the rising incidence of child impairments, and began to get curious and ask questions. Not surprisingly, I found that a large number of the children on my caseload who were referred for physical, mental, social or academic problems were high users of entertainment technology. I became alarmed when I began to realize that the education and health systems were possibly misdiagnosing children who had technology addictions, with mental and behavioral disorders. While the child indeed may have exhibited developmental delay, obesity, mental illness, aggression, adhd, or learning problems, in many cases these impairments were *caused* from technology overuse. Missing the salient causal factor misdirects the intervention. As many of these diagnostic categories assigned to 21st century children are psychiatric in nature, many of these children also receive psychotropic medications (stimulants, anti-depressants, anti-anxiety, sedatives, and/or anti-psychotics). The role of technology overuse as a causal factor for this observed phenomenon of over diagnosis and medication, has neither been recognized nor addressed during my time as a school-based therapist, and goes largely ignored by health and education professionals even today.

The health of children is a determinant of societal success, and 21st century children are far from healthy. Research reported in this book will reveal a shocking 14.3% of Canadian children have a diagnosed mental illness (Waddell, 2007), and many are taking adult psychotropic medication that has never been proven effective or safe with adults, much less tested on children (Zito, 2000). 30% of Canadian children are developmentally delayed (Kershaw, 2009), and 15% are obese (Tremblay, 2007). Half of grade eight children do not have the literacy skills necessary to secure a job (National Center for Education Statistics, 2010). Soaring child aggression is creating behavior management problems in classrooms and at home (Small, 2008), which has been implicated in the recent classification of media violence as a public health risk by the medical and psychiatric community in the United States (Huesmann, 2007).

It gets worse. Chronic high adrenalin and dopamine transmitter levels from video game use, cause further stress to human physiology (Small, 2008). At 7.5 hours per day average use of entertainment technologies (Kaiser Foundation, 2010), children are not participating in activities they need to optimize their growth and success. Addicted to technology, socially isolated, unintelligible speech, maldeveloped, sensory hyper-vigilant, failing in school, depressed and anxious, taking "neurotoxic" psychotropic medications...the sustainability of our children is truly now in question. The American Academy of Pediatrics recommends children use no more that 1-2 hours per day of entertainment technologies, and the National Association for Sport and Physical Education recommend children participate in 2-3 hours per day of unstructured play. Studies show that "green space" and exercise improve cognition, attention and learning abilities. What can parents and teachers do to reverse this worrisome trend? Could it be so easy as to just tell our children to go outside and play?

Readers will find that *Virtual Child: The Terrifying Truth About What Technology Is Doing To Children* contains not only facts related to the impact of technology overuse on children, but also contains a detailed, clear and concise plan for counteracting this impact. Bringing together key players through the formation of teams including parents, teachers, health professionals, government, researchers and technology production corporations, will form the foundation for change. Employing numerous effective and efficient strategies and initiatives proposed in this book, to be enacted in home, school and community settings, will form the operating system for change. Bringing the fast tracked "technology train" back to the station at this point in time is integral for forming evidence based action plans needed to move forward in a responsible manner.

I've developed a concept termed *Balanced Technology Management* where homes, schools and communities work together to manage balancing technology use with critical activities children need to grow and succeed. This concept is described in detail in the third section of this book and suggests children, parents, health and education professionals practice abstaining from all forms of technology for one hour per day, one day per week, and one week per year. During these times without the influence of technology, participants are invited to explore alternative activities to build child performance skill and confidence.

Our best "bang for our buck" and first step will be found in the education of children through implementation of media awareness programs in school-based settings. I believe in the power of the child, and if children can experience greater health and productivity by balancing activity with technology in school-based settings, then they will be empowered to take these concepts home and demonstrate them to their family and friends. With our foundation teams working to employ *Balanced Technology Management* initiatives that support a new way of being for our children, and our children taking these concepts home, we can enact the changes needed to ensure sustainable futures for all children.

SECTION I

Problems Resulting from Technology Overuse – The Perfect Storm

Growing a child is like building house – it's all about the foundation. If the foundation of a house is faulty, through poor design or use of inferior materials, the house will sustain life long and permanent problems. If the foundation of a developing child is faulty, through not receiving essential elements at critical times during their development, the overall growth and long term outcomes of the developing child will be permanently altered. If the foundation for a house or a child is insufficient or missing enough critical elements, the house and the child reach a point where no intervention will keep them from falling down, or collapsing on themselves. This is where we are at today. We are experiencing a world where whole families, through overuse of technology, are collapsing all around us. Increasing incidence of aggression, obesity, attention problems, learning difficulties, family conflict, sleep disorders, sexual promiscuity, and behavior problems are now becoming the norm for the new millennium child. We have unconsciously created fertile conditions for *The Perfect Storm*, posing a threat to the most vulnerable members of society – our children.

When planning for a baby, parents think about their dreams and aspirations for their child, where they will go to school, and who they will be when they grow up. Expectant parents have all these wonderful plans of spending time together as a family, cuddling on the couch, going for walks, reading silly books, playing peak-a-boo games. Then the baby is born. There are diapers to be changed, feeding problems, crying and lack of sleep. All of a sudden the parent's world is turned upside down, with limited guidance on how to cope. While the actual job of parenting hasn't really changed in the history of humankind, new age technology has offered parents many devices that offer the continuous opportunity to escape the rigors of parenting. The "virtual babysitter" is replacing parenting at an alarming rate. 25% of young infants now have televisions in their bedrooms because parents can't be bothered to rock them to sleep. Young toddlers are increasingly handed iPods, iPads, cell phones and a plethora of DVD's, video games and television programs. Of course, all these devices are cleverly marketed as "educational" by the producers as an attempt to alleviate parental guilt.

Technology has rapidly become an accepted interface between the parent and child, alienating families and breaking the fragile bond that is life sustaining and integral to healthy development. This distance between parent and child caused by technology, quickly evolves into an impassable chasm, culminating in a wave of attachment and behavior disorders that the health and education systems misinterpret as mental illness. Connection between parent and child forms the "blueprint" for their development, for the very foundation of their being. Alone and neglected, in the absence of parents, the *new age* child has no choice but to disconnect from humanity and connect to technology. This disconnection between parent and child caused by technology overuse is the most significant destructive factor ever witnessed by humankind, and will not only damage the foundation for the developing child, but also cause irreversible damage to humanity, and not just for the short term, but forever.

In addition to human connection, touch and movement are two other critical factors for the "blueprint" used to build healthy and strong foundations for child development. Touch helps infants, toddlers and young children to feel safe and secure in the boundaries of their developing and changing bodies. Movement is essential for not only cardiovascular health and prevention of obesity and diabetes, but also in the development of coordination and strength necessary for eventual attainment of literacy. Sensory deprivation and motor delays are but a few of the developmental problems we are seeing in today's children resulting from technology overuse. Technology has imposed dramatic and irreversible changes on our children, even children as young as one year of age. By the time these children enter high school, they are immersed in a virtual culture that consumes and pervades every aspect of their lives, forever altering the ways in which they communicate and form relationships.

We live in the "Me Generation", a world where children get what they want and adults seem to have forgotten what it means to parent, or are simply too tired to make any rules that create guidelines for children. Without rules or boundaries, children either run around aimlessly creating havoc and chaos, or worse yet, retreat into an isolated and lonely world of their own. Whether they are demanding and expecting immediate gratification, or are anxious and scared from being neglected, these new age children are growing up without the necessary challenges that create *inner drive*, a force essential for the survival of our species. Not giving children on a daily basis the essential elements they need to form foundations for healthy development, is resulting in conditions ripe for a cataclysmic disaster, *The Perfect Storm*.

Frustrations of a High School Counselor

The proliferation of sites like Facebook and YouTube, although good in some ways, have reduced the natural boundaries or taboos that existed before, that limited the degree and amount of harmful things that immature adolescents could inflict upon one another.

High school has always been subjected to a certain amount of gossip among its student population, but now any gossip gets spread like wild fire. Some very hurtful things get expressed because kids are saying such things in the privacy of their own homes or elsewhere. It's a lot easier to say mean things if you are not face to face with the target of your criticisms. As a result, cyber bullying is on the rise.

Facebook and internet use have also eliminated adult supervision, so that younger and younger students are navigating daily in a technological world of their own making. I believe that this has contributed greatly to the early sexualization of our adolescents. They are exposed to sexual matters at a younger and younger age and I feel that they (although teens would not admit it) are being pressured to become sexually active sooner than they are ready. I believe that the proliferation of pornography on the internet and kids' access to it, have contributed to reducing sexual activity to a very superficial, materialistic level. Of course, not all teens view sex in this way and families can have an impact on the values that are being formed in their children. But I believe that more and more teens have a very flippant and superficial attitude towards their sexual lives.

This superficial approach, can lead to a certain level of despair and alienation amongst teens. In our fast paced world of instant gratification, nothing is really very special any more. This has perhaps led to an increase in teenage depression and suicidal ideation.

As a high school counselor, when I do get the chance to speak to students about an emotional issue, I have had to request (more frequently in the last 2 years) that they do not text message in the middle of our conversation. Texting "etiquette" is something new that teens need to learn, it appears. It seems that students do not know how to have a face to face conversation anymore; they are so out of practice. Many students seem to feel comfortable only when interacting indirectly through the use of some technological tool.

I have seen students sitting side by side on a bench in our school having a conversation with one another by texting on their cell phones. In other words, they are talking to each other with their fingers rather than with their voices. They make no eye contact and are unaware of body language.

Are our children forgetting how to talk to one another? I'm not sure, but I am starting to think that this may be happening. And it is altering our human experience, and not for the better, I may add. Our human interactions are being speeded up on a daily basis and the quality of our lives and relationships are being reduced as a result. As a society we are becoming more and more superficial and fickle, and the beauty, joy and satisfaction of being deeply connected to others in our world is being seriously altered by the rising use of technology.

Can anyone appreciate a sunset anymore, or do we have to watch a video on YouTube (with an inspirational soundtrack added on) to able to be awed by the wonder of it all?

Deborah Alain, Art Therapist and High School Counselor, British Columbia

Technology - Everyone Doesn't Have To Do It

This section of *Virtual Child* is written to help readers begin to understand the complexities of the *direct effects* of technology overuse on the developing child, through exploration of the research literature. This information will prepare parents, health and education professionals with the necessary framework with which to plan how to better manage technology and lessen its detrimental impact on children. The information covered in this section will provide readers with essential skills to accurately analyze *who, what, when, where, why* and *how* technology impacts on different children in different environments. Readers will also learn about the numerous and pervasive *indirect* or secondary effects that technology has created in a child's home, school and community settings. This information will enable readers to be experts in the knowledge required to ensure children participate in activities they need to optimize their development and academic success, and help them to prioritize child engagement in these activities over technology. Technology is neither good nor bad, and when determining "how much is too much", every aspect of technology and its myriad of effects on children must be carefully and knowledgably taken into consideration.

A Mom at War

Parents today are just a grain of sand and the whole world is a tidal wave of electronics pushing against them. If your child doesn't have a cell phone/iPod/Nintendo then you are a bad parent because "everyone else" has one.

My daughter's school got an educational grant to pay for an X-Box in her classroom. Really? There isn't anything else you can use to motivate her? She rides horses and loves dogs and reading... she loves being social with other children.

People use technology because they are LAZY and it's EASY. When my daughter uses the computer or her DSI she will barely respond to anyone talking with her. My friends all agree. I am so grateful that my neighbors all insist on the kids playing outside every day. They ride their scooters, climb trees, play sports and make up their own games together.

But at SCHOOL they shorten recess to 15 minutes. They bring in an X-box and when I ask how is THAT educational I'm told "Well, I'm just afraid of how left out your child is going to feel if she can't play and everyone else can". But because she didn't have the "techie toys" to play with on the bus, she TALKED with the other kids. They know she loves dogs and her bus driver knows she loves music. How are people going to communicate if their attention spans get shorter and shorter as the world around them moves faster and faster? I know I can't get rid of technology but this is WAR and I'm holding the line.

Wendy Grande, Mom of a daughter with autism, Pennsylvania

Chapter 1

Who, What, When, Where, Why and How?

When a child has a health or learning related issue, this child may first be referred into the health or education system for problems that initially appear to have nothing to do with technology overuse. Many of the referrals I receive are for sensory or motor related issues, or for problematic behavior. As I only see children in their homes with one or both parents present, I have a unique opportunity to observe not only family interactions, but also their relationship with technology. It is only when I take a technology usage history from both the parents and the child that I really begin to see some of the possible contributing factors to the child's presented problem. For example, I was referred to a young 6 year old girl whom I'll refer to as "Sally" by her school resource team for apparent sensory integration impairment and behavioral problems. Sally was termed by her teachers as "high energy" and reportedly had great difficulty concentrating on tasks in the noisy classroom setting. While academically bright, Sally's teachers stated that she had few friends and they termed her "socially immature". When I first saw her in her home environment, Sally had just arrived home from school and appeared quite excited yet nervous at my presence. Sally repeatedly asked to go down to the basement to play video games, and required considerable coaxing to stay upstairs and participate in my assessment. Sally's parents reported that Sally did use "a lot" of technology, and her mother stated that they had been trying to "cut down" but unsuccessfully. Upon further questioning, I became aware that Sally's parents had no idea of the ramifications of technology overuse, nor did they understand how this overuse could be contributing to Sally's presented problems.

When addressing whether a child's problems are partially or wholly related to technology use, the first step is for parents, health and education professionals to gain evidence-based information regarding current technology impact research. When reviewing this research, it is important to "tease out" the many different parameters of technology, such as what type of technology is the child using, the age of the child, and possibly the frequency and duration of technology use. Analysis of these technology parameters allows a much clearer picture of this child's usage patterns. It is also important to examine not only the *direct* impact of this technology on the child, but also the secondary or *indirect* effects of this technology use in the child's home and school environments. It is only upon closer examination of this information that one begins to see the profound impact technology has had on children's lives. Making decisions using research based evidence, and applying this research through thoughtful analysis of all the different factors that come into play, results in decisions that have long reaching implications for improving child health and academic performance. If this procedure is not adopted, parents, health and education professionals are left to make decisions based on their belief systems, technology marketing, or worse still the concept that "everyone is doing it".

One statement that I frequently hear teachers say is that technology enables children to learn. While this statement might contain a shred of truth for some students, there are others who should never use technology, and there are specific situations where technology use *disables* the learning process. In order to assist adults to make informed decisions regarding technology use by children, I've listed a number of factors which need to be considered. These factors will assist in deciding *who, what, where, when, why,* and *how* children should or shouldn't use technology. Unfortunately, waiting for research to address these questions may not be the most expedient way to gain guidance regarding child technology use, at least not in our lifetime.

The technology explosion has hit our family, health and education systems so hard and so fast, that they haven't even begun to recognize the enormity of the problems facing young children as a result, much less develop initiatives to counteract its devastating effects. We are currently just witnessing the tip of the "technology iceberg" so to speak, with many more issues festering under the surface. Existing research on the impact of technology on children is fraught with many challenges, least of which is to create reliable and reproducible data that isn't antiquated before it gets published. By the time the results of research studies on technology hit our mainstream media, the data is already incomplete as some new technological device has been developed. Or, child technology usage rates have risen incrementally during this research duration. In light of *who, what, when, where, why* and *how*, what could we possibly tell our teacher who commented that technology enables learning? How could we apply research principles to either prove or disprove this statement? Relying on educational technology company marketing literature is neither evidence-based nor wise, and may prove to produce more harm than good.

As 75% of children have technology in their bedrooms, it is virtually impossible for parents to know how much technology their child is using (Kaiser Foundation, 2010). It is therefore imperative that health and education professionals also interview the child when taking a technology history, as well as provide the parents with the following *Technology Screen*. The *Technology Screen* can be filled out by parents as a handout from health and education professionals. The screen is designed to obtain an accurate technology usage history for the child in question, and is recommended to be a routine part of any teacher or clinician's history taking of the child. I designed this technology screen to be filled out on a daily basis for one week duration. The *Technology Screen* should include not only technology usage information from the child in question, but also include the parent(s) and sibling(s) usage of technology as well. This family technology usage history is important during treatment planning, as studies indicate that child usage patterns simulate that of their parents (Vanderwater, 2005)

Analysis of the results of the *Technology Screen* can then be incorporated into the child's overall intervention plan as deemed appropriate by the health and education-based teams. As the American Academy of Pediatrics and the Canadian Pediatric Society both recommend that children limit technology use to 1-2 hours per day, comparing the results of the *Technology Screen* to expert recommendations would shed light on whether indeed this child's physical, mental, social or academic problems in question might in part or whole, be attributed to technology overuse. The results of the *Technology Screen* should also serve as a guide toward appropriate and effective interventions for overuse and addiction. Researchers might want to consider inclusion of the *Technology Screen* in future research in order to delineate whether or not technology use is an independent or dependent variable in their research design.

Technology Screen

Today's children are exposed to a variety of electronic media technology. This exposure could be detrimental to their developmental well-being based on the frequency, duration and intensity of the technology use. Bedroom technology prohibits parents from accurately knowing how much technology their child uses. *Technology Screen* is designed to provide information to guide you toward assisting your family to manage a balance between activities your child needs for growth and success, with their use of technology. "Technology use" is defined as television, movies, computer, cell phone, video games, iPods and any other electronic devices. There are additional grids for other family members.

Name: _____ Does your child use technology in their bedroom?   Yes / No

How much does your child use technology...	Mon	Tues	Wed	Thu	Fri	Sat	Sun
in the morning?							
in the afternoon?							
during dinner?							
after dinner?							
one hour before bed?							
in the middle of the night?							

Total hours per week, divided by 7 = average hours per day of technology use _____

Name: _____ Does your child use technology in their bedroom?   Yes / No

How much does your child use technology...	Mon	Tues	Wed	Thu	Fri	Sat	Sun
in the morning?							
in the afternoon?							
during dinner?							
after dinner?							
one hour before bed?							
in the middle of the night?							

Total hours per week, divided by 7 = average hours per day of technology use _____

Name: _____ Does your child use technology in their bedroom?   Yes / No

How much does your child use technology...	Mon	Tues	Wed	Thu	Fri	Sat	Sun
in the morning?							
in the afternoon?							
during dinner?							
after dinner?							
one hour before bed?							
in the middle of the night?							

Total hours per week, divided by 7 = average hours per day of technology use _____

Chapter 2

Determining Guidelines for Child Technology Use

To ensure child safety when using technology during this time of uncertainty, I have designed the *Technology Guidelines* to help parents, education and health professionals determine the impact of technology use on children. These *Guidelines* should be used in conjunction with the previously outlined *Technology Screen*. These two tools, when used together, will provide adults accurate information which can be then used in the management of technology in home and school settings. Achieving balance between activities children need to grow and succeed and technology use, will ensure sustainable futures for all children.

Technology Guidelines

Technology Parameters

Who – age, developmental level, academic ability, diagnostic category.
What – *platform:* television, movies, video games, internet, iPads, cell phones, iPods, other.
What – *content:* violence, sex, education, comedy, sports, reality, sitcom, cartoon, nature.
When – during meals, before bedtime, in the car, on family holidays.
Where – home, school, car, restaurant, friends, family homes and community.
Why – *child:* escape, socialize, bored, control, build self esteem, educate, addicted.
Why – *parent:* pacify, attachment replacement, placate, reward, low self esteem, educate.
How – duration, intensity, frequency, transportability.

▼

Direct Effects

Physical – obesity, developmental delay, disrupted sleep, cardiac stress.
Mental – difficult behavior, anxiety, depression, adhd, autism, addictions, medication, chronic fatigue.
Social – aggression, isolation, communication, lack of empathy, early sexuality, truancy, few leisure pursuits.
Academic – inattention, learning disability, poor performance (grades), illiteracy.

▼

Indirect Effects

Home – attachment disorders, family violence, divorce, foster care, medication side effects, poor socialization, failed partnerships.
School – increased testing, reduced recess, increased diagnosis, fiscal collapse from technology expenditures, elimination of teaching printing and book reading, police presence, drugs/alcohol use, weapons, school drop out, expulsion, lack of university pursuit.
Community – reduced interest in parks, recreation and community events, fear resulting in increased focus on police and security presence.

Technology Guidelines - Practical Applications

In order to demonstrate how the *Technology Screen* and the *Technology Guidelines* can work together, I've detailed a case history of a child I recently assessed and to whom I provided interventions. The *Technology Screen* and the *Technology Guidelines* helped me to create an accurate picture or profile of the child in question. Analysis of this child's profile sheds much needed "light" on whether indeed this child's physical, mental, social or academic problems in question might in part be attributed to technology overuse. An intervention plan was then easily determined as deemed appropriate in conjunction with the parents and other health and education-based teams. This child's profile could also serve as a guide toward appropriate and effective interventions for technology overuse and addiction. This sample case study typifies how the *Technology Screen* and the *Technology Guidelines* could be used to guide professionals toward "best practices" in their treatment of children, and ensure the "real" underlying problem is addressed and treated appropriately.

Technology Guidelines Case Study

"Cody" was a 7 year old boy who was referred by his parents at the request of his school based team for behavioral problems and sensory and motor impairment. Cody was diagnosed with autism at 4 years of age, and at age 6 was recommended stimulant medication which his parents had refused. Motor skills assessment determined Cody was developmentally delayed by two years in fine/gross motor skills, and observations indicated his expressive and comprehensive speech was equivalent to that of a 4 year old. Cody's printing, reading and numerical literacy was also at a 4 year old level. Sensory assessment indicated Cody was hypersensitive for auditory and tactile stimuli, and that he had difficulty registering sensation that was new or changing. Cody had no friends, and did not initiate social interactions at school with his class mates, nor at home with his parents. Cody's technology usage patterns at home were "unrestricted" with usage of approximately 10 hours per day during the week, and up to 18 hours per day on the weekend. These statistics were determined from information obtained from both Cody and his parents. Cody's parents stated that due to his severe behavioral responses to rules, they were prevented from imposing any restrictions regarding Cody's technology use. As Cody predominantly used an iPad technology platform, Cody was able to access technology any time he wanted to, from any room in his house, as well as in the car, restaurants and in extended family and friend's homes. Cody played mainly violent video games, but also watched cartoons and old sitcoms which he had viewed repeatedly.

Direct Effects Report

Cody presented as moderately overweight with low trunk tone and poor motor coordination. He demonstrated a rigid body posture and slight "trembling" of his arms and hands during video game play, and for up to a half hour after play was stopped. Cody's parents reported he was frequently up during the night, as he had difficultly getting to sleep and could only stay asleep for durations of up to 3 hours. Cody's parents recounted they were both very tired at night and needed get up early to work during the day, so they found it easier to not restrict Cody from technology during the night. Both Cody's parents and school staff report that Cody had difficultly controlling aggressive "outbursts" and state that Cody did not appear to show remorse or empathy for his peers or teachers if he hurt them. While Cody was able to communicate his needs at home with his parents through gestures, he was withdrawn and non-verbal in the school setting. Problems with socialization and aggression toward his peers apparently limited Cody from participating in a classroom learning experience. School staff report Cody spent up to 4 hours per day in the special education room doing his "work" either on a XO computer or his iPad platform. Cody was rewarded for completion of his educational work on the computer with the use of his favorite video games.

Indirect Effects Report

Cody's parents state they had little or no "real" relationship with their son, and often used texting or email as their only form of reliable communication with him. While Cody's parents were receiving couple's counseling, they both stated their home environment is "dismal" and would likely separate soon. Cody's parents and teachers reported that children did not want to play with him at school, or come to his home due to his aggression. Cody's teacher relayed that Cody's energy was always either sleepy and zoned out, or hyper and charged, rarely reaching the "zone" needed to pay attention and learn. Due to poor classroom participation and aggression problems, Cody's school provided his curriculum on an XO computer which he could use in any location. Based on these reports from the school, Cody's pediatrician had diagnosed him with adhd and recommended stimulant medication. Since provision of the XO, Cody has been refusing to go to school, choosing instead to do his "work" at home on his XO, requiring one parent stay at home. Cody's Mom told me that on occasion she has left Cody at home by himself for periods of 4 to 5 hours. Cody had been expelled from school on three occasions in the past year, reportedly for causing bodily harm to other children, and on one occasion to his teacher.

Interpretation

While readers may think this is an exceptional case history, it is one I'm quite familiar with and have witnessed aspects of on numerous occasions. Using the *Technology Screen* and the *Technology Guidelines* helped me to determine that many of Cody's problems originated from his technology overuse. His delayed development, obesity, sleep disorder, aggression, decreased sociability, adhd, learning problems, illiteracy and lack of empathy, could all be contributed to some degree to high levels of technology use, much of which contained media violence. If I had not performed the *Technology Screen*, and consulted the *Technology Guidelines*, I likely would have attributed all of Cody's issues to his diagnosed autism, which may in part originate in the disconnection he experiences with his parents.

Intervention

Luckily for Cody, his parents were very interested in pursuing technology reduction, and even agreed to advocate for technology restrictions in his school environment. Based on their comments, Cody's parents seemed to *know* that many of his issues were related to technology overuse, but stated that no one had ever described to them the extent of detrimental effects on children. Once they were aware of the facts, Cody's parents showed what can only be termed "enthusiasm" in moving forward on a path of technology reduction. Unfortunately the school was not as convinced that Cody could reduce his use of technology, without causing an escalation in aggressive behavior. The school reported that reduced use of technology would require increased teaching assistance for the education of Cody, which the school stated they neither had the staffing or funding to put in place. So, the focus was home technology management.

Prior to setting technology restrictions for Cody, I counseled the parents that the first step in technology awareness and reduction, was for the both of them to evaluate their own technology use patterns. Unless the parents could cut down on their usage, they could not be available for the necessary interaction and human connection required for Cody. Human connection in the home environment is essential for the formation of social relationships at school. The parents were told that it was imperative that Cody develop new interests and skills to replace his pursuit of technology, and that they needed to help him in this process. Cody's Dad stated that he had always wanted to take Cody skiing, a sport he had not pursued since his university days, and teach Cody to ride a bike. Cody's Mom thought that since Cody likes to eat, and she likes to cook, that they could take a cooking course together. Discussion ensued regarding creation of "sacred" times without technology during which the family would go for walks or play structured games. A technology schedule was placed on the fridge where each family member would schedule their weekly technology use, as well as a balance of healthy activities that did not require technology.

Outcomes

Cody was able to cut down his home usage from 10 to 4 hours per day during the week, and 18 to 6 hours per day on weekends over the course of a 12 week period. Through use of printing worksheets produced by the *Move'in Program*, Cody increased his printing output speed by 2 years, and began to initiate his homework independently at home. Cody's Dad taught him how to ride a bike, and allowed him to independently ride 2 blocks to the local store to get supplies for the family home. Cody's parents did not bring up marital separation again with me, and looked happier and healthier than when I first met them. Cody began to make eye contact and initiate communication with me, and reportedly began to make friends at school. Cody's family started family "theme" nights, where they created a repeating weekly schedule of family activities. While Cody still used over the recommended expert limits of technology, the amount he reduced his technology use, greatly improved his mood, grades and relationships. I was relieved that Cody had avoided the administration of stimulant medication through technology reduction and connection-related activities with his parents.

Technology Guidelines for Children with Disabilities

As an occupational therapist I am acutely aware that many children with severe disabilities benefit from the use of technology. Many children with cerebral palsy who are non-verbal actually use technology to speak. These children should obviously receive unrestricted access to their technologies. Concern arises when a child is provided technology to compensate for the lack of teaching, as has been my experience on numerous occasions. Another example of inappropriate use of technology is with young non-verbal children with autism, who are being provided devices to compensate for speech. While this might be an appropriate intervention when the child is older, while the child is young, attachment formation, sensory processing interventions, and lots of movement based activities should be performed. It is only after all attempts at eliciting voluntary speech have been exhausted, that technology should be considered. To default to technology use as a first intervention for an output modality, deprives these children of a lifetime opportunity to interact with other human beings.

Words from a University Professor, who also has autism

I am concerned that too many of the nerdy, geeky Asperger-type children are getting so addicted to video games that it is difficult to get them to do other things.

I had a lot of special interests when I was young and my fixation on cattle chutes became the basis of a successful career. If video games had been available in the 1960's, I would have become an addict. That would have led me nowhere because I did not have the math skills to learn video game programming and make a career in video game design.

There are two kinds of kids who get addicted to video games. There are the ones who can turn it into a successful career in the video game industry, and the ones like me who do not have the math skills to do game programming. A video game fixation would have led me nowhere fast. Instead, I got obsessed with cattle chutes and that was turned into a successful career.

In my talks and books, I recommend that video game playing be limited to one hour a day. When I was a child, I was allowed to have one hour a day to spin things and tune out.

You may wonder, why are video games so additive? When I was little and loved watching cartoons, there was something about all the rapid movement that just sucked me in. Since no video games were available in the 1950's and 60's, I spent hours playing with parachutes made from scarves, toy airplanes, and kites. Many of my flying toys I invented. When I grew up, I ended up in a career where I designed and made things.

In conclusion, I think video game playing should be limited to one hour a day. I do not recommend banning it. Forbidden fruit causes many problems. Kids need to be encouraged to do lots of different things. I have lots more ideas in my books, "Thinking in Pictures" and "The Way I See it."

Dr. Temple Grandin, world renown speaker and author, Colorado

Chapter 3

Technology Usage Statistics and Expert Recommendations

Head-Downers, Screenagers, and Appholes

I was instructing kids on how to draw a cartoon cloud. I asked the kids if anyone had taken an airplane flight. One 11 year old said he had. I asked him what color the clouds were when he looked down on them through the window of the plane. He said he never looked out of the window, because he was paying his PS2 through the entire flight.

I had a kid come up to me and tell me that her father knows me. I asked his name, but it wasn't familiar. When I asked her how he knew me, she said he looked me up online. To this kid, that equates to her dad "knowing me". Ouch!

On a bus ride home form my hospital work I met a well dressed well spoken young man in his 20's who was making points about people being overly connected to technology. He told me about meeting an attractive young woman on the bus, having a great conversation with her, and suggesting they meet sometime to continue their conversation. She told him to "Look me up on Facebook." That was her virtual alternative to actually sitting down with this guy she met on the bus."

Steve Broshihan, Resident Cartoonist at a Children's Hospital, NY

The following statistics have been obtained from research data and government websites, and reflect the extent of technology usage by North American children up to the year 2010. As this area of study is rapidly changing, I recommend that readers also refer to child health websites which constantly update their information. I have a research-based *Fact Sheet* on my website zonein.ca that is organized by topic with alphabetical research references. *The Center for Media and Child Health* is a researched-based health organization affiliated with Harvard University located at Boston Children's Hospital. This center has an extensive research database and categorized information for parents, teachers and researchers regarding child technology usage statistics. The following research statistics were chosen to support the information presented in *Virtual Child*, but by no means are a complete research list:

- A recent study by the Kaiser Foundation in 2010 found that North American children use an average of 7.5 hours per day of entertainment technology (television, video games, movies, internet, cell phones, iPods, and other devices). This figure does not include any educational based technologies, which in some schools could be as high as an additional 4 hours per day.
- As children frequently use 2-3 devices at a time, the total amount of technology usage rises from 7.5 hours to 11.0 hours per day.
- While many parents find these figures shocking, they need to consider the fact that over 75% of children have technology in their bedrooms, making use largely unsupervised (Rideout, 2003).

- This Kaiser Foundation study found that only 30% of children have parents who set any rules at all regarding technology use, and those parents who do set rules, have children who use 30% less.
- One out of every four infants aged 0 to 2 years have televisions in their bedrooms, and "baby TV" now occupies 2.75 hours per day (Christakis, 2009).
- Infants are spending far more time restrained in "bucket" seats, originally intended for use in cars, resulting in an increased in infant "flathead" (flattening of the back of the skull) by 600% over the past 5 years (Jennings, 2005).
- The toddler population is using an average of 4.5 hours of technology per day (Rideout, 2003).
- Active Healthy Kids Canada gave Canadian children a grade of D for inactivity, citing television and video games as the primary cause (Active Healthy Kids Canada, 2008).
- Sedentary lifestyle is resulting in one in three children with developmental delay (Kershaw, 2009), and one in six children with obesity at school entry (Tremblay, 2007).
- 50% of households have the television on all day, as do a growing number of restaurants, cars, and even physicians' waiting rooms (Nielsenwire, 2009), causing a dramatic reduction in parent-child communication (Vandewater, 2005).
- Parents who allow the television to be on all day communicate 80% less with their children, a drop from 941 words per hour to 200 words per hour (Christakis, 2009).
- Child behavior problems have become unmanageable in both home and school settings, with 14.3% of Canadian children receiving a mental health diagnoses (Waddell, 2007).
- Many health professionals are now questioning this apparent "diagnostic frenzy" (Kershaw, 2009), as the medical and psychiatric professions have failed to find any genetic or biological cause for *any* mental illness to date (Breggin, 2008).
- Continued escalation of diagnostic procedures seems not only unwarranted, but also may be harmful. 15% of elementary aged children are now taking some form of psychotropic medication, such as stimulants, anti-depressants, anti-anxiety, and anti-psychotics (Zito, 2002).
- This psychotropic medication use in children continues to escalate unchecked by the medical profession, despite mounting research indicating psychotropic medication is not effective (Raine Study, 2010), in many cases has proven harmful (Baughman, 2009), and in some cases is actually fatal (Jensen, 2002, Vitiello, 2009).
- To date, there are no *long term* research studies for psychotropic medication use by children, with the adult research indicating increased risk of suicide and/or violent behavior (Breggin, 2008).
- Media violence has been categorized as a "public health risk" in the US due to copious research documenting causal links to aggression in both the toddler and child populations (Anderson, 2008; Christakis, 2007; Huesmann, 2007).
- The incidence of both bullying and cyberbullying continue to escalate (Anderson, 2009), as violence in school settings reaches an all time high (Vancouver Sun, 2010).
- 50% of children referred into the medical system for child behavior diagnosis, are referred by their "disease spotter" teachers (Sax, 2008).
- Children who use greater than the recommended 1-2 hours per day of technology, have a 60% rise in psychological disorders (Bristol University, 2010).
- As media violence causes child aggression, one has to wonder if education and health professionals are unknowingly medicating child behavior associated with technology overuse (Rowan, 2010).
- Declining child literacy continues to plague educators throughout North America. One third of children entering the school system will drop out of high school, failing to achieve job entry literacy (Kershaw, 2009).
- Every hour of technology used per day is associated with a 10% increased risk of

attention problems (Christakis, 2007).

- Children who overuse fast paced technologies such as video games, are "pruning" their brains to not access their frontal lobes, known for executive function and impulse control (Small, 2008, Murray, 2006).
- Delayed, obese, uncommunicative, mentally ill, aggressive, adhd and illiterate, one third of our new millennium children may actually end up dying before their parents, raising the question "Are 21st century children sustainable?" (BBC News, 2002).
- The American Academy of Pediatrics in 2004 issued a policy statement indicating that children 0 to 2 years of age should not be exposed to any form of technology, and elementary-aged children, should be limited to 1 to 2 hours technology per day.
- In 2010, the Canadian Pediatric Society echoed these concerns and endorsed these aforementioned guidelines. These limits include both entertainment and educational technologies in the form of cell phones, internet, television, video games, movies, iPods and any other electronic devices.
- Today's *Virtual Child* is using on average four times the recommended amount of technologies, with grave and long reaching results.

Direct Effects - The Impact of Technology on the Developing Child

In 1970 - 0% of children were on psychotropic medication. In 2008 – 15% of children are on some form of stimulant, anti-depressant, anti-anxiety, sedative or anti-psychotic medication. What has changed between then and now?

The salient answer is vastly increased technology usage.

Cris Rowan, Pediatric Occupational Therapist and Author, British Columbia.

The following section profiles the impact of technology on the developing child, and is divided into two parts:

1. *Direct* effects of technology on child physical, mental, social and academic performance.
2. *Indirect* effects of technology on homes, schools and communities.

Chapter 4

Physical Impairments

From We to Wii... Child Development Is No Game.

No matter what new gaming platform technology production corporations develop, use of technology is largely sedentary. Even if children are swinging a 200 gram "virtual" baseball bat (a feather compared to the weight of a real bat), they are still inside staring at a screen and not developing social play skills. Technology overuse is the salient reason why children of the new millennium are less physically active than they have ever been in recorded history. This inaction by children results in dire consequences to their physical development and overall health. A 2009 study by Paul Kershaw, a pediatric researcher with the University of British Columbia's *Healthy Early Intervention Partnership* program revealed that secondary to a sedentary lifestyle, one in three Canadian children will enter school developmentally vulnerable, with delays in fine and gross motor tasks, communication ability, socialization, and cognition. Many of these children will go onto fail their grade four and seven regulated exams, resulting in failure to graduate from high school.

The *Canadian Institute of Health Research* in 2004 referenced child sedentary lifestyle as a causal factor for the current 15% child obesity rate. Resolving child developmental delay and obesity has many child health care experts and researchers scrambling to develop initiatives, many of which are actually quite scary and misguided. Groups of child care experts in England and Ireland are advocating for removal of obese children from their homes due to "parental neglect" (Viner, 2010). The thought that we would remove children from their homes, in advance of offering quality parent education and support to reduce the technology use which caused the obesity, is outrageous. While the health ramifications from child developmental delay and obesity are likely to bankrupt the health governments, and immediate measures are definitely needed, labeling well meaning parents as "neglectful" if they have an obese child is pointing the finger at the wrong person.

The *American Heart Association* in 2010 reported increasing incidence of cardiovascular disorders in children, secondary to rising rates of obesity, and pointed to sedentary lifestyle and poor diet as causal factors. *The Center for Disease Control* in 2010 reported health care providers are identifying more and more children with type 2 diabetes, a disease usually diagnosed in adults aged 40 years or older. Children are sedentary largely due to technology overuse, yet this fact is rarely referenced by child health researchers, and hence, recommendations are often misguided and limited. Worse still is that parents are not receiving correct and useful information about the salient causal factor for sedentary lifestyle – technology use. Children are not just sitting around *doing nothing*, they are sitting around because they are intensely engaged in video games, or passively watching television. Why don't researchers report and profile this critical information? Parents cannot act if they don't know all the facts.

Media also are to blame in the failure to accurately inform parents regarding the ramification of technology overuse. The *British Broadcasting Corporation* reported in 2004 that a young boy spent an entire day kneeling down playing computer games and consequently required hospital treatment for a blood clot in his leg due to poor circulation. No further information was offered regarding expert recommendations for technology use by children (obviously this child had exceeded these limits), nor was there any information about the possible link between technology overuse and cardiac problems. In fact, there was no information at all, just that this child was hospitalized.

Current day media style appears to go for "shock value" in their reporting of events, and rarely follows their story with related additional information or helpful suggestions. The average parent reading this article about a child being hospitalized from a blood clot as a result of playing video games, would likely conclude that this would be a rare occurrence, one that their child would not be succumb to. In 2002 the BBC reported that Andrew Prentice, a professor at the *London School of Hygiene and Tropical Medicine* stated that due to the results of a sedentary lifestyle and consequent obesity, cardiovascular problems and diabetes may result in the 21st century generation being the first generation to not outlive their parents. If the BBC had linked these two pieces of crucial information (prolonged technology use causing a blot clot, and sedentary lifestyle causing children to die before their parents), possibly parents would be more informed and more likely to act to restrict their own child's technology use.

The following sections profile the direct impact technology is having on children's physical development, and includes topics of developmental delay, obesity, visual and auditory system impairment, sleep deprivation, chronic stress, irreversible brain damage, and cell death.

Developmental Delay

While *sedentary lifestyle* is frequently referenced in the research literature as having a *causal* relationship to developmental delays, *technology overuse* by young children is only referenced in the research literature as being *associated* with developmental delays (Hamilton, 2006; Zimmerman, 2007). This failure of researchers to state the underlying causal factor for the rise in developmental delay misleads parents, as well as health and education professionals down the path toward ineffective interventions. I repeatedly read about initiatives to increase movement activities to address delayed development, yet nothing about reducing technology use. Parents, daycare and preschool providers, and educators should be informed that their intervention and prevention initiatives for developmental delay should include technology management and reduction. To not be aware of this salient fact is jeopardizing the health and well being of not only millions of young children, but also their families.

An example of early delays in developmental milestones is the rising incidence of infant "flat head", which has increased 600% in the past 5 years (Jennings, 2005). Infant flathead is caused from infants spending long periods on their backs, and as the skull is still "soft", prolonged back laying results in a flattened area on the back of the infant's head. This same study cites that two-thirds of physiotherapists in the United States report increasing incidence of "low tone" in infants, generally caused by sedentary lifestyle. Researchers failed to site television watching in cribs, bucket seats, and strollers, as contributing factors for infant flathead. With the rise in the use of television in infant's bedrooms, one can only guess that sedentary television watching must play a significant role in infants continuous lying on their backs. Another question to be asked regarding the rise in infant flathead is whether technology addicted parents might be neglecting their children by leaving them restrained in front of televisions? There is a lot of parental education to be done in this area, and accepting that technology is a huge part of family life, the professional's role should now include that of taking a routine *Technology Screen*, with appropriate guidance given to families regarding technology reduction strategies.

This rising evidence of developmental delays in young children has prompted France to recently ban its broadcasters from airing television shows aimed at children less than 3 years of age (CBC News, 2008). In the United States, the *Federal Trade Commission* pressured the *Disney Foundation* to offer full refunds on all of its Baby Einstein DVD's citing "false advertising" regarding claims of improved cognition and speech (New York

Times, 2009). Accurate information regarding the detrimental impact of technology on developing children has been slow to circulate amongst the general public. This is best evidenced by the pervasive and continued escalation of both entertainment and educational technologies in the home, daycare, pre-school, and school-based settings.

To date, I have presented over 200 workshops to parents, educators and therapists regarding child developmental delays, and repeatedly received comments referencing an astounding lack of information by both health and education professionals in this area. I repeatedly tell parents and professionals that any time spent in front of technology is detrimental to child development, and should be minimized at all cost. Actually, minimizing technology use in the home, daycare, and elementary setting would save billions of dollars to both governments and societies combined.

Obesity

The *World Health Organization* reports that globally, more 21st century children will die from conditions related to *obesity* than to *starvation*. Television and video game use is evidenced to be a factor accounting for 60% of childhood obesity, which is now considered a North American "epidemic" by physicians (Tremblay, 2005; Strauss, 2001). A report from the *United States Centers for Disease Control and Prevention* states that child obesity rates continued to escalate from 2007 to 2009 despite increasing attention being paid to the health costs and problems associated with excessive weight. This report goes on to state that as of last year, 72.5 million Americans, or 26.7 percent, are obese, a jump of 2.4 million in two years, and reports that the rate of obesity exceeded 30 percent of the residents in nine different states. Again, this obesity research identifies only sedentary lifestyle and the eating of "junk" foods as causal factors, and rarely mentions technology use as the major reason why these children are sedentary. While most parents are aware that the watching of commercials for junk food raises desire and eventual use of these non-nutritious foods, and actually "brands" young children to buy specific products, it is not carefully spelled out to these parents that reducing the use of technology would contribute to a reduction in obesity.

As stated previously, climbing obesity rates in European countries have led a team of child health experts to recommend placing obese children in foster care, citing that parents of obese children are negligent in allowing their child to become obese (Viner, 2010). By neglecting to identify child technology overuse as a causal factor in rising incidence of child obesity, these child health experts are subjecting whole families to what might be an unnecessary and unwarranted traumatic and catastrophic event – the loss of their child to an already overloaded foster system, who probably *also* over use technology. I was told by a foster parent at one of my workshops that she was informed of a requirement for foster parents in British Columbia to have a television in their homes, as it "calms" children. I was unable to find this requirement in any of the provincial government online literature for foster parents, and therefore, it may have been just a misinterpretation or a local regulation. Regardless, what are we doing telling foster parents that instead of forming meaningful connections with their foster children, they should *disconnect* and *reconnect* them to a device? Can you imagine a situation where a child was removed from their home citing parental neglect because the child was obese, and then the child was placed into a home that promoted technology use?

The failure of governments in choosing not to mention technology overuse in their obesity public health prevention campaigns is again irresponsible and quite frankly, confusing. Why wouldn't they? Risk warnings could easily be mandated to be placed on all technology products stating "This product will increase the risk of child obesity", including suggestions for responsible use. Profits aside, technology production corporations have an obligation to "Do No Harm" to our young children. Choosing to not educate parents regarding the potential detrimental effects from the use of their product, places technology production corporations in a legally liable position.

Media fails the general public miserably each and every time they run a story about child obesity, without mentioning the salient causal factor – technology, along with helpful suggestions to parents for reduction of use. We live in a world of short, incomplete stories that offer catastrophic bits of information, without ever exploring causality or solutions. Have we really succumbed to this level of disinterest in the health of our children, or are we simply all too fragmented ourselves to make the necessary connections?

Visual and Auditory System Impairment

Prior to the advent of technology, young children were engaged in long periods of outdoor play, consisting of nature-based and benign, visual and auditory stimuli. During play, children would visually focus on both short and long distance targets, while also rotating their heads in different planes of movement. These types of movements resulted in children being able to coordinate the muscles of both eyes, as well as develop excellent visual acuity. Children looking at nature in three dimensions allowed their visual systems to develop a variety of perceptual skills, such as depth, visual figure ground, and visual memory, all of which are useful when learning how to print and read. Exposure to a three dimensional visual world, especially through the lens of nature, is integral in the development of the visual system, which children use exclusively when learning.

Historically, children exposed to nature were able to accurately distinguish individualized, specific sounds, against the backdrop cacophony of all the sounds of nature together. As they strained to hear a waterfall, or buffalo grazing in the grass, nature's world helped the child's auditory system develop its innate ability to register, modulate and discriminate different sounds. Children who are able to discriminate different sounds, are also able to filter out the "surround noise", such as other students in a classroom, and be able to tune in to hear what the teacher was saying.

Today's world of intense visual and auditory stimulation (from technology over use) is far different from nature's past. Long duration exposure to loud, visually graphic, and often violent electronic stimuli may be forever changing the ways in which young children's visual and auditory sensory systems develop (Christakis, 2009). Gone is the three dimensional world, replaced by a fixed distance, two dimensional screen. Gone is the "wide arc" visual scanning and rapid head movements, necessary for optimal visual development. Gone are the quiet yet intricate sounds, replaced by chaotic, loud and assaulting auditory stimuli. Gone is visual and auditory learning as we once knew it, replaced by complex and competing stimuli we know very little about. As educators instruct students primarily using the visual and auditory sensory systems, further knowledge regarding the impact of technology overuse on these developing systems would seem warranted, especially with the escalating use of computers as teaching tools in schools. There is likely also a limit to how much chaotic and intense visual and auditory stimulation a young child's developing neurological system can experience without causing irreversible damage. As a child's ability to attend, comprehend and interpret visual and auditory stimuli is a requirement for optimal school performance, the effect of long duration chaotic exposure through television, video games, computers and cell phones on that child's ability to learn in a school setting requires immediate research attention.

When studying the developing visual sensory system, Dr. Christakis, a pediatric researcher with the University of Washington found in 2009 that exposure to television in infants activates what he terms an "orienting response". This orientating response to visual stimuli causes the infant to stare at the television screen for prolonged periods. Dr. Christakis warns parents that this response is often misinterpreted as "interest", and therefore parents could be thinking their infants are *choosing* to watch television, when really they are under the influence of a primitive visual reflex. Reports from India and Europe indicate that children with photosensitivity have increased incidence of seizures when using video games (Singh, 2001; Kasteleijn-Nolst, 2002). Many children with autism experience photosensitivity (Baron-Cohen, 2010). With growing rates of autism, risk warnings regarding video game use and possible seizure activity might be warranted, and technology restrictions put in place in both home and school settings.

Sleep Deprivation

During workshop presentations, I increasingly receive reports from teachers and school-based therapists about the problem of sleep deprivation, with students falling asleep in class. Sleep deprivation has been found to have profound consequences on a child's ability to think and reason, as well as their emotional state. As 75% of children have an electronic device of some sort in their bedrooms, this technology use is rarely supervised by parents and has consequent impact on their quality and quantity of sleep. Paavonen found in a 2006 study that technology use is causally related to a reduction in sleep duration, with a disruption in sleep and wake cycles. This study also highlights the effects of having the television on all day in homes as being detrimental to the sleep and napping cycles of very young infants and toddlers. New York Magazine in 2007 featured an article "Snooze or Loose" which described the results of research performed by Avi Sadeh, a professor at Tel Aviv University who found that a reduction in as little as one hour of sleep per night, for a 3 night duration, lowered elementary student's scores on achievement tests by two full grades. Children who are up late at night playing video games, or who wake up in the middle of the night because they can't sleep and default to playing video games, are not going to be as alert or productive in the classroom setting the next day, and may even fail school as a result.

Adolescence research has shown that not only does sleep deprivation effect school productivity, but it also has an effect on mood. A study by the *National Longitudinal Study of Adolescent Health* found that adolescents whose parents allow bedtimes of midnight or later are 24% more likely to be depressed, and 20% more likely to express suicidal ideation than adolescents whose parents set bedtimes of 10 PM or earlier (Gangwisch, 2010). This adolescent research raises the question "Could sleep deprivation be a contributing factor to the rising levels of mental health diagnosis in children?" If so, why aren't parents informed that overuse of technology may cause sleep deprivation, and that if their child is sleep deprived, this may negatively impact on academic performance. Removal of technology from children's bedrooms could have a profound impact on academic performance and behavior.

At the very least, parents should receive comprehensive information on the impact of technology on child mental health and academic performance in order to make the best decisions regarding technology use for their child. The 2010 Kaiser Foundation Study reports that only 30% of parents set limits and rules regarding technology use, resulting in their children using 30% less technology (Kaiser Foundation, 2010). If the resolution to many of the problems that result from technology overuse, can be as simple as informing parents and helping them to set rules, maybe the problem is not as big as we think!

Chronic Stress

Gary Small, a neuroscientist with University of California and author of the book *iBrain: The Technological Alteration of the Human Mind* reports that exposure of children to violent media content has been shown to cause increases adrenalin and cortisol. While release of these substances is a normal response of the sympathetic nervous system to stress, what happens when a young child's body is in a *chronic* state of arousal from prolonged use of violent media? High and prolonged levels of adrenalin and cortisol are known to impact negatively on the body's cardiovascular and immune systems, as well as result in a condition known as "chronic fatigue" where the body is actually depleted of adrenalin and cortisol. We know that stimulant medication in some children has a negative effect on their heart, and also that many children who have been diagnosed with adhd and are taking stimulant medication also overuse technology (Raine ADHD Study, 2010). Can we deduce then that stimulant medicated children with adhd who also overuse technology are at *increased risk* for cardiac problems? This area needs immediate research, and suggests that stimulant medication should NOT be used in children who overuse technology.

In occupational therapy clinic settings, children who overuse technology have described physical sensations of body shaking, rapid heart rate and shallow breathing. An area requiring further research would be to investigate whether technology overuse is creating chronic stress states in children, a condition that if proven true, could have long term and devastating consequences to child physical and mental health. In very young children, I have observed full body muscle contractions and tremors while they play video games, almost as if their body wants to *move*, yet they are actively working to *restrain* or *constrain* this movement, resulting in increased stress states. Upon first observing this phenomenon in young children, I was struck with the thought that in infant, toddler and elementary aged child populations, these children's bodies may not actually know that what their brain is experiencing isn't "real". These young bodies may be actually experiencing what could be termed a "fear response" to what the brain interprets to be frightful stimuli. Could young children exposed to prolonged and high levels of media violence consequently go on to develop a form of post traumatic stress disorder? This is another area that requires immediate research.

Irreversible Brain Damage

Dr. Small also reports in his book *iBrain* that researchers who studied the developing neurological system of children who overuse technology for prolonged periods, found that during video game use, these children were not activating the *longer* (and therefore slower) neuronal tracks to the frontal cortex, but rather defaulting to the use of *shorter, faster* neuronal circuitry. Dr. Small reports that the developing brain's response to this "disuse" was for it to "prune" or stop neuronal transmission to the frontal cortex, which is the brain's epicenter for executive function, formation of goals, and impulse control. To put this concept in evolutionary terms, our frontal lobe is what distinguishes human beings from animals further down the food chain. To lose the function of our frontal lobes, is actually reversing evolution – to some degree. Imagine a generation of children who no longer are connected to their frontal lobes. These children would be out of touch from their source of higher level thinking, distanced from important concepts such as morality, ethics, and wisdom. Instead, humans would fall back on their more basic cognitive functions: calculations, day to day routines, and mundane tasks. What will our world look like when the majority of the population is using less and less of their brain?

This landmark research should challenge every education professional to think very carefully when they continue to term technology "educational". While an immediate result may be slightly faster reading speeds, or improved ability to add and subtract, the long term outcomes must be taken into consideration when whole school systems make the decision to download a full year's curriculum onto an XO or TeacherMate, and tell parents that this device will enable long term and comprehensive learning for their children. While some high school aged students will benefit from use of computers in school-based settings, or at least those who go on to use computers in a work-place setting upon graduation, not all students need computers and some students who are over users of technology, may be sustaining irreversible brain damage from their use.

I am frequently challenged on this apparent "illusion" that computers are "learning" tools by teachers. While there may be some shred of evidence that a computer program will improve a specific aspect of a child's learning, the detrimental effects of being sedentary, as well as decreasing access to frontal lobes, may actually eliminate any benefits. What if the studies on educational technologies, which are usually performed by the technology production company themselves, used children who were under-users of technology, and therefore had adequate functioning frontal cortexes? Could the results of these studies then be applied to children who over-use technology? I doubt it.

What is striking about these studies is that after a one year period of reduced technology use, these children had not *reformed* neuronal connections to their frontal lobes. This finding indicates that children who are exposed to increasing amounts of technology may be irreversibly damaging their brains, and causing damage to the specific area of the brain dedicated to learning. The obvious question is "How will our education system teach to children who have limited or no executive function and no impulse control?" We quite simply *do not know*.

Cell Death

Recent media coverage by *The National Post* in October, 2010 regarding unknown, long term risks associated with school-based Wi-Fi (wireless internet) use, poses many questions. Historically, the use of *intermittent* microwave radiation has been around since the 1940's. What is new, and has received limited and only short term research, is *continuous use* of microwave radiation, also referred to as extremely low frequency electromagnetic fields (ELF-EMF) in the form of wireless internet, cell phones, televisions, and computers with children in both home and school settings.

Recent events in Ontario schools have brought concerns regarding the dangers of ELF-EMF to the forefront, and prompted parents to request schools to provide a liability waiver for their children if the school uses wireless internet. With the rapid escalation of technology use by children, comes also the need for establishing polices to ensure safety through *responsible use*. While many technologies are not harmful in and of themselves, the frequency, duration and intensity parameters of microwave radiation must be taken into consideration when determining whether (or not) a specific technology is safe. Children are now using an average 7.5 hours per day of entertainment technology at home. Exposing children to additional "educational technology" use in the school-based setting may prove to be not only detrimental to achievement of literacy and learning, but also harmful to children's physical and mental health.

Recently released research in 2010 from the *Department of Biophysics, Faculty of Medicine* in Cukurova University, Turkey indicates exposure to ELF-EMF, causes oxidative cell damage and cell death in rats. This study reports that in humans, oxidative stress is involved in many diseases including atherosclerosis, Parkinson's disease, heart failure, myocardial infarction, Alzheimer's disease, schizophrenia, bipolar disorder, fragile X syndrome and chronic fatigue syndrome. Another study reports that cell phone use results in brain tumors (Khurana, 2009). Yet – the overuse of these technologies by children in both home and school settings continues to escalate unchecked, even with very young children. I was recently told by teachers that the British Columbia Education Ministry is encouraging the placement of computers in kindergarten classrooms for pre-reading skill training. This initiative not only lacks supporting evidence, but based on current research, will likely result in irreversible long term harm to child health.

The National Post reported in October, 2010 the Ontario School Board stated that wireless internet use in schools poses no harm. The article goes on to state that Magda Havas, a professor in the *Centre for Health Studies* at Trent University in Peterborough, Ontario said other forms of microwave exposure — particularly cell phone towers — have been linked to cancers, heart problems, sleeping problems, skin conditions and short-term memory loss. Children are also more likely to be vulnerable, due to weaker immune systems and because their bodies are still growing. "It is possible, and I think it is even probable, that this exposure will have an effect on children," Havas said. Professor Havas issued an open letter last year saying she was "increasingly concerned" about Wi-Fi and cell phone use at schools. "It is irresponsible to introduce Wi-Fi microwave radiation into a school environment where young children and school employees spend hours each day," Havas wrote. Statistics show young children absorb much more radiation than older children and adults because of their thinner skulls. It is a public health issue, insisted Havas, and should at least be taken as seriously as the threat of West Nile virus.

Chapter 5

Mental Illness and Psychotropic Medication

Observations by a Child Mental Health Professional

Our rate of adolescent, and younger, CO (constant observation) patients has dramatically increased over the past few years. These are kids with emotional issues that sometimes have a physical counterpart. They must be constantly observed because of the threat of them hurting themselves.

In a conversation with a senior nurse recently, I heard an interesting opinion. She thought, along with doctors she works with, that a lot of these kids have not developed the skill of coping with stressors and instead turn their frustrations back on themselves. There is a possibility that the overuse of electronic stimuli has robbed them of the human interaction needed to develop coping skills in general, and particularly with other humans. They lack the "rough and tumble" play needed for blowing off steam and instead suffer an overload of stress. It is a very sad thing to witness, and a major burden on the nursing staff.

One psych doctor suggested that a good 15-minute walk would be worth a normal dose of mood-altering drug that these kids unfortunately end up on.

Steve Brosnihan, Children's Hospital, Road Island

A 2010 study at Bristol University found that children who use greater than the recommended 1-2 hours per day of technology, have a 60% increase in psychological disorders. Continuing to label behaviors related to technology overuse as "mental illness", and prescribing psychotropic medication rather than unplugging the technology, is nothing short of unconscionable. While there are literally thousands of behavior modification approaches available, the propensity to diagnose and drug children as a first line choice of treatment for problematic behaviors could potentially be viewed as "abuse" and may be placing the education and health professional at risk for eventual legal action. When we know that exercise and access to nature improve behavior, why don't we just instruct students outside on the playground? It's important to understand why the education and health systems have adopted this "diagnose and drug" model, in order to then try to reverse some of its momentum and power.

Psychiatric Times in 2009 reported that recent changes from a "categorical" to a "dimensional" model in the upcoming *Diagnostic and Statistical Manual for Mental Disorders, Fifth Edition (DSM-V)* to be released in 2013, has "Opened the flood gates for increasing diagnosis of children", reports Dr. Allen Frances who was chair of the DSM-IV Task Force. Dr. Francis stated that this "paradigm shift" is premature, as there is still not even ONE biological test ready for inclusion in the criteria sets for the DSM-V for any mental illness. What this means is that all mental health diagnoses are based on the child's behavior, not biology. Increasing numbers of experts in the field of child psychiatry are now questioning whether there even is a biological component *at all* in child mental illness (Breggin, 2008; Baughman, 2006). A discussion paper prepared by Charlotte Waddell in

2007 for the British Columbia *Healthy Child Development Alliance* showed that 14.3% of Canadian children between the ages of 4 and 17 have a diagnosed psychiatric disorder (Waddell, 2007). In the United States 13% of survey respondents 8 to 15 years of age who participated in the 2009 *National Health and Nutrition Examination Survey* reportedly met criteria for at least one of the following mental health disorders in the past year: generalized anxiety disorder, panic disorder, eating disorder (bulimia and anorexia), depression, adhd, and conduct disorder. We can't forget autism. Statistics from the *Centers for Disease Control and Prevention* report 1 percent of United States children now have autism or another autism spectrum disorder.

Parents are besieged by a plethora of well meaning health and educational professionals with a growing list of mental diagnoses designed to describe their child's confusing and difficult to manage behavior. In a study of 491 physicians in Washington D.C., almost half of the diagnoses of adhd in their patients had been suggested first by teachers (Sax, 2003). Christine Phillips, professor at the *Australian National University Medical School* reports that teachers have now taken on the role of "disease spotters" and "sickness brokers" for adhd, and is concerned regarding what she terms the "Escalating infiltration of the pharmaceutical corporations into the school system". Yet – are these children really mentally ill and in need medication, or are they suffering from inactivity, exposure to violence, isolation and possibly busy, neglectful parents?

The following information profiles the direct impact technology is having on children's *mental health*, and covers the following areas: mental illness and behavior diagnosis; medicating technology addictions; social isolation, addiction, and suicide; evolution of adhd and autism; diagnosis, medication and therapy; and the dangers of medicating children.

Mental Illness and Behavior Diagnosis

Parent time spent connected to various forms of technologies is disconnecting them from forming healthy, primary attachments with their children. This parent-child disconnection is possibly a major contributing factor to the reported increased incidence of mental diagnoses. A recent study revealed that 20% of parents did not know how to "play" with their children, and one third of parents found play "boring" (Guardian News, 2010). The results of this study indicate that far less time is spent in meaningful communication and connection between parent and child, often with grave consequences. Parental time that could be spent in conversation, play, and other "non-care giving" type of activities with their children, has been eroded due to the constant pressure on parents to check their emails, text messages or phone calls. I have received reports from both school and daycare staff that an increasing number of parents provide their children with cell phones for the purposes of unrestricted contact between parent and child throughout their school day. While they might be on their cell phones when dropping their child off at daycare, resulting in a stressed and teary "good-bye", these same parents are phoning their child 10 minutes later to do a "check-in" to see how they are doing. Another study showed that parents who stay in touch with their university aged children using social networking (texts, email, Facebook), have children who indicate more loneliness, anxious attachment, as well as conflict within the parental relationship, than children who's parents stay in touch in person or by phone (Gentzler, 2010). While we like to think we are more "connected" using social networking, the reverse is unfortunately the case.

Many areas where family conversation used to flourish, such as on holidays, in the car, at the dining room table, and before bedtime, have all been invaded to some degree by technology. As the dining room table is slowly replaced by the big screen, an epic shift in family structure and operating systems is rapidly taking place, a shift that may result in irreversible changes to family relationships, and in some cases, cause detrimental effects to child mental health. It has recently been reported in the press that parental addictions regarding involvement in online gaming and avatar programs, have resulted in child neglect charges and even child death. Two parents were recently arrested and charged with neglect causing bodily harm when the social ministry in the United Kingdom discovered they were neglecting their two young children, choosing instead to raise two children on a *Second Life* avatar program (Telegraph UK, 2010).

Traditionally, the family physician's role was to treat child physical injuries and illnesses, not difficult behaviors, attachment disorders, and learning difficulties associated with child and parent technology addictions. As physicians and pediatricians generally see clients in office-type settings for short durations, and are not able to view the child or parent interactions in the home or school setting, information with which they base their mental and behavioral diagnoses of children may be quite restricted. As it is currently not a requirement for health professionals to screen or assess children for technology overuse or technology addiction, this important contributing factor to child behavior and learning ability is often missed.

Are We Medicating Technology Addictions?

A Pediatric Neurologist's Views on Depression

We read of "...new bouts of illness," and of "...the fact that depression is an episodic disease." The fact of the matter is that everyone on earth, everyone alive, will experience countless episodes of depression, of greater or lesser severity, and innumerable occurrences of all other emotions as well—all of them constituting our entirely normal barometer of life and living. These normal emotions are not to be ignored or suppressed as psychiatry would have us do, to believe, instead, that such feelings are "illnesses," "diseases," or "chemical imbalances." Nor are they to be erased with psychiatric pain pills. They must be acknowledged, understood and acted upon if we are to find a happier, more successful day. Such fictions and contrivances are the stuff of the marketing campaign of the psychiatric- pharmaceutical cartel, and are meant only to deceive and to sell psychiatric drugs— "chemical balancers" for "chemical imbalances"-"diseases" of the brain. There are no such things. Psychiatrists are no longer patient advocates, they are one-dimensional "pushers" to anyone and everyone, an arm of the pharmaceutical industry.

Dr. Fred Baughman, Pediatric Neurologist and Author, California

The recent rise in incidence of behavior problems and learning difficulties in children, is resulting in what Dr. Kershaw termed a "diagnostic frenzy", often associated with an alarming use of psychotropic medication (Mandell, 2008; Ruff, 2005). Between 1991 and 1995, prescriptions for psychotropic medications in the 2 to 4 year-old toddler population, as well as in children and youth, tripled (dosReis, 2005; Goodwin, 2001; Zito, 2000; Zito, 2002). Eighty percent of psychotropic medication for children is prescribed by family physicians and pediatricians (Zito, 2003), and twenty-eight percent to 30% of children receiving psychotropic medication are on multiple medications (dosReis, 2005). Limited evidence guiding appropriate dosing, and inexperience in the documentation of long-term effects of these prescriptions in children, may mean that these children undergo unquantified risks (Rosack, 2003; Kirsch, 2004; Thomas, 2006). Who are all these children, and why are they in so much psychological pain that they are supposedly requiring medication?

A comparative study of children diagnosed with adhd who were on stimulant medication showed a 10% decrease in growth rate (height and weight) when contrasted with children diagnosed with adhd who were not receiving stimulant medication (Swanson, 2007). A study performed by researchers from the *Government of Western Australia, Department of Health*, report reduced academic performance and increased risk of heart malfunction in children who receive adhd medication, and found that children taking stimulant medication were more likely to be performing *below* their age level at school by a factor of 10.5 times (Raine ADHD Study, 2010). This study also reported that a child's heart function may be affected by long-term stimulant use and may remain affected even after stopping medication. Additional researchers are concerned regarding the correlation between stimulant use and cardiovascular risk in children (Vitiello & Towbin, 2009), and indicate immediate attention should be directed to non-pharmacological behavior interventions for the treatment of child behavior and learning disorders. Yet – a recent study from the University of Michigan found that in 7 out of 10 cases, stimulant medication was the ONLY treatment offered to parents of children diagnosed with adhd. North America prescribes a staggering 95% of the world's stimulant medication (Breggin, 2008). When England and Australia have discontinued the use of psychotropic (including stimulant) medication in children, United States and Canadian education and health professionals need to ask themselves "Why are we the only two nations in the world with adhd"?

With this unprecedented rise in child mental diagnosis and use of psychotropic medication, concurrent with the rise in child use of technology, the routine use of the child *Technology Screen* by all health and education professionals would be warranted. Child health researchers may also want to consider mandatory use of *Technology Screens* in their health and academic research, in order to accurately assess the impact of technology use on child physical, mental, social and academic status. How could researchers, in this day and age of technology, accurately design research parameters without a technology screen? This technology screen should act as a preliminary step to guide mental or behavioral diagnosis, and certainly be required prior to any use of psychotropic medication. Based on the results of the technology screen, a technology "unplug" trial may be warranted. Termed "Unplug – Don't Drug", the child and all family members would undergo removal from all forms of technologies (except those required for school or work) for a period of three months (Rowan, 2010). Only after this 3 month "unplug" trial and consequent reassessment, would a mental or behavioral diagnosis be assigned. If other countries are restricting use of psychotropic medication, so should the United States and Canada. Section III of *Virtual Child* details numerous alternatives to the use of diagnosis and psychotropic medication for problematic behaviors in children.

Social Isolation, Addiction and Suicide

While no one can argue the benefits of advancing technology in today's world, many children are spending their days alone in dark rooms. Engagement with technology for long durations, in a virtual and often violent world, is disconnecting children from the world of physical play and meaningful human interactions. The effects of social isolation are sadly numerous, and have far reaching consequences. A German nationwide survey in 2007 and 2008 of 44,610 ninth graders indicates that 3% of male and 0.3% of female students were diagnosed as *Video Game Dependent* (VGD) and spent significantly higher amounts of their time alone than non-VGD controls. Addiction was defined as an obsession with playing electronic games to the point of sleep deprivation, disruption of daily life and a loosening grip on reality, depression and with drawl when not playing. This survey reports that *Video Game Dependency* is accompanied by increased levels of psychological and social stress in the form of lower school achievement, increased truancy, reduced sleep time, limited leisure activities, and increased thoughts of committing suicide (Rehbein 2010).

Difficulty identifying feelings, higher dissociative experiences, lower self esteem, and higher impulse dysregulation are associated with higher incidence of internet addiction (DeBerardis, 2008). Adhd was found to be the most associated symptom of internet addiction, followed by impulsivity (Yen, 2008). Internet addicts were found to be lonelier and have lower self-esteem and poorer social skills than moderate users (Ghassemzadeh, 2008). Video game addiction can be statistically predicted on measures of hostility and poor academic achievement (Shao-I, 2004). 12% of boys and 8% of girl video game players exhibit pathological patterns of play, and fit the DSM IV category of addiction (Gentile, 2009). This same study also showed that pathological gamers are twice as likely to have adhd.

Whether it is indeed an addiction, or possibly just a "dependency", *identifying* that a child has a problem with overuse of technology is imperative, if education and health professionals are going to be able to help them. Following is a *Technology Addiction Questionnaire* designed to assist adults in raising awareness regarding the level of technology addictions in children, whether at home or school.

Technology Addiction Questionnaire

The term "technology" refers to use of any or all of the following devices for entertainment purposes (as opposed to education or work): television, video games, internet, movies, cell phones, iPods or any other electronic device.

		Yes	No
1.	**Tolerance**: Your child watches the same amount of technology as they used to, but frequently requests more.		
2.	**Withdrawal**: Your child can't imagine going without technology.		
3.	**Unintended Use**: Your child often watches or uses technology for longer than allowed time limits.		
4.	**Persistent Desire**: Your child has tried to stop using technology, but can't.		
5.	**Time Spent**: Technology takes up almost all of your child's leisure or play time.		
6.	**Displacement of Other Activities**: Your child sometimes watches or uses technology, when they should be spending time with family or friends, doing their homework, or going to bed.		
7.	**Continued Use**: Your child keeps watching or using technology, even though they know it isn't good for them.		

Total number of "yes" answers _____

If you answered "yes" to 3 or more questions, your child is addicted to technology.

Personal Technology Reduction Plan for Parents

I, _____ plan to reduce the amount of technology use from my current _____ hours per day down to _____ hours per day.

Instead of watching or using technology, I plan to do the following activities with my child (circle or add new ones): biking, climbing trees, playing sports, baking, sewing, playing cards and/or board games, playing outdoor games with my child's friends, plan a party, do volunteer work, visit elderly people, garden, do chores as a family, build something, take something apart, or...........

_____

_____

Xiao Yi was thirteen when he threw himself from the top of a twenty-four story tower block in his home town, leaving notes that spoke of his addiction and his hope of being reunited with fellow cyber-players in heaven. Xiao Yi's suicide notes were reportedly written through the eyes of a gaming character (Play TM News, 2005). The underlying causal factor for addictions is failure of the primary attachment system between primary parent and child (Flores, 2009), a concept discussed in further detail in Section II. As parents connect more and more to technology, they disconnect from their children. In the absence of a healthy relationship with their parent, children will form unhealthy relationships and attachments to technology. Unfortunately, these attachments are not life sustaining, and through risky and destructive behaviors, or isolation and depression, theses children may not survive.

The Evolution of Adhd and Autism

Just a thought... it was interesting when I was working up in Fort Ware that out of 300 people, with far less exposure to technology and far more boredom, we had no autism.

Jessica McKerrow, Special Education Teacher, British Columbia

I have always wondered why children from First Nations communities do not "get" autism. I have heard numerous theories, but have never come across any valid research that provides insight into this dilemma. Having worked in Northern communities myself, I have always been struck by the amount of time First Nations community members spend outside, even in the harshest conditions. This closeness to nature, and strong sense of community, may make aboriginal people somehow immune to autism.

Michael Waldman, an economist with Cambridge University found in 2006, that areas with high autism density are also areas of high rain fall. His study showed that high rain fall is associated with significantly higher amounts of television watching in children. While it is a long stretch to say television causes autism, there are some interesting facts in this study that indicate at the very least, a routine *Technology Screen* by education and health professionals is warranted. If indeed these children who have autism watch more television than children without autism, then interventions and support to manage balanced use of technology with other activities would be indicated.

Dr. Nahit Motavalli Mukaddes, a researcher and child psychiatrist from the Netherlands in 2000 studied 15 children who were misdiagnosed with autism. After 3 months of their parents receiving weekly psycho-emotional therapy treatments, all 15 children who were previous diagnosed with autism, were consequently re-diagnosed with reactive attachment disorder. Dr. Mukkades reported that the children in this study watched 7.26 hours of television per day, and 33.3% of this time these children were alone, constituting what was termed by Dr. Mukaddes as "neglect" with consequent "pathological care" administered by the parents. Directing autism research away from exhaustive and expensive biological, neurological or genetic investigations, toward looking more closely at environmental and family-based factors, is imperative when considering the escalating rise in autism, and the prevalent technology overuse by parents and children.

While science has continued to fail to "discover" the cause of either adhd or autism, we do know that both of these disorders are characterized by attachment difficulties. Dr. Gabor Mate', a renown speaker on adhd and author of the book *Scattered Minds: A New Look at the Origins and the Healing of Attention Deficit Disorder*, refers to adhd as an "attunement disorder" (Mate', 2007). John Merrow, a well respected teacher and author of *Below C Level: How American Education Encourages Mediocrity and What We Can Do about It* references adhd as "attachment deficit disorder". Addressing the accompanying attachment disorder in children with adhd and autism would likely serve to result in improved functioning in these children as in the Muddades study. If we do not thoroughly investigate the environmental and nurturing aspects behind the exponential rise in adhd and autism, we are doing a disservice to parents everywhere. If these two disorders, and child mental illness in general, had their origins in primary attachment formation, then we could finally begin to direct funding and focus on where we can help the most, by supporting the nurturing parent. Regardless of whether this information is "true" or not, supporting the primary attachment system between parent and child is always a good intervention. How could it not be?

Another similar area of impairment found in both children with adhd and autism is an inability to self-regulate their sensory states. 94.4% of adults and 69% of children with autism demonstrated sensory processing dysfunction on the *Sensory Profile* (Crane, 2009; Baranek, 2006). The greatest differences were reported on the under-responsive/seeks sensation, auditory filtering and tactile sensitivity sections. Researchers found in 2007 that children with adhd have increased tactile defensive behaviors (Parusch, 2007), also observed when children are deprived of touch (Montagu, 1972). These inabilities to regulate incoming sensory information often result in "sensory overload" states of sympathetic *fright, flight* and *fight* (Tomchek, 2007). This impairment can result in a child reporting feelings or perceptions of "pain" when exposed to specific types of auditory or touch stimuli, necessitating treatments to either protect or desensitize the adhd and autistic child's central nervous system. Those familiar with the work of Dr. Temple Grandin may remember her use of deep pressure techniques to induce calming. Dr. Grandin, a professor in the area of animal behavior with Colorado State University, and author of *Animals in Translation: Using the Mysteries of Autism to Decode Animal Behavior* has autism, and through the use of a self made "squeeze" machine, was able to desensitize her tactile system and induce a sense of self regulation and calm (Grandin, 2006).

To better understand the evolution of the adhd and autistic child, as well as to better understand their tactile and auditory sensory systems, we need to look at what has happened in our technology evolving world over the past decade. For hundreds of thousands of years, human beings were engaged in heavy work, and sensory stimulation was nature-based and fairly benign. Chopping wood, hauling water, plowing fields...listening, looking and smelling nature. Recent advances in technology and transportation have resulted in a physically sedentary human body that is bombarded with chaotic and complex sensory stimulation. While schools are reducing recess and gym time, homes are increasing television, internet and video game time. Continued budget cutbacks have resulted in reduced organized sports at recess, as well as overcrowded classrooms with subsequent "caged animal" symptoms in children (anger, anxiety, chewing, and depression).

Biologically, children's nervous systems need excessive and intense touch and movement to develop properly; swinging, hanging, jumping, pushing and spinning are all necessary movements for development of child sensory and motor systems. If these systems don't develop properly, processing in the higher level auditory and visual systems are affected as well. Remember merry-go-rounds, tall swings, climbing ropes? Remember our parents kicking us outside after school and all day on weekends and summer? We need to wonder what we are doing to children by providing them with a deficit in the movement and touch sensory systems, while also providing them with an auditory and visually sensory frenzied existence. Combined with busy and detached parents, are these conditions ripe for development of autism and adhd? What will be the consequences for these children if we continue to escalate technology use?

Our world is not adapting as well as we would hope to the consequences of a sedentary yet frenzied lifestyle. For children who don't have adhd or autism, I have observed one in three primary classroom children have attention problems limiting their ability to learn, and one in four students have printing delays. Many of the referrals I receive for children are for sensory impairments, most frequently for impairment in the tactile and auditory sensory systems. Should we just save the education and health systems a whole lot of time and money and just diagnose all children with adhd and/or autism? While this statement holds a fair degree of sarcasm, it also holds a looming and scary truth – that the education and health systems working together have rapidly turned North America into *One Nation Under Therapy*.

Child behavioral diagnosis, medication, and therapy – Who really benefits?

Record levels of *new* child diagnoses have overwhelmed both the education and health care systems, burying professionals in a pile of referrals, wait lists, reports, and education plans. Are North American children really "sick" and "learning disabled", or have the education and health systems unwittingly created a self serving monster? Is the prolific categorization of children actually helping the children, or is it instead serving an industry of health and education professionals, causing an eventual bankrupting of the governments and destruction of childhood as we once knew it? What is wrong with the *New Millennium Child*, and how can society help get them back on track toward a more healthy and sustainable future?

A systematic review of evidenced based research, and the asking of pertinent questions, is imperative in order for health and education systems to establish polices that will protect children, and address some of the questionable child care practices performed by health and education professionals today.

- When we know that North American children use 7.5 hours per day of entertainment technology per day (Kaiser Foundation, 2010), and that those who use more than 1-2 hours per day have a 60% increase in psychological problems (Bristol University, 2010), *why aren't health and education professionals teaching parents how to reduce the use, instead of recommending diagnosis and medication?*

- When we know that every hour of television and video game use by children per day increases adhd risk by 10% (Christakis, 2004), *why are the education and health care professionals choosing adhd diagnosis and use of stimulant medication as a first line intervention?*

- When we know that child access to "green space" for 20 minutes a day significantly reduces adhd (Kuo, 2002), and 20 minutes of cardio exercise per day significantly increases attention (Ratey, 2008), *why are 15% of the elementary population in North America taking stimulant medication to control behavior (Zito, 2002)? Why not just recommend increased outdoor play?*

- When current research shows psychotropic medications are no more effective than a placebo, disrupt growth hormone causing brain atrophy and a 10% reduction in height and weight, and result in cardiac sudden death in 1-2% of children (Breggin, 2009), *why are professionals increasing use of psychotropic medication with society's most vulnerable children?*

- When research shows stimulant medication use results in a ten fold decrease in academic performance (Rhine ADHD Study, 2010), *why is it still prescribed at all?*

- When psychotropic medication has proven to be "neurotoxic" to children's brains, causing serious side effects that are often misinterpreted, resulting in increasing the dosage, changing the drug, or adding an additional medication, *why is psychotropic medication use becoming the norm rather than the exception?*

- When research indicates 50% children on adhd stimulant medication get depressed and are prescribed antidepressants, and 50% develop obsessive compulsive disorder, which looks like a manic phase of bipolar disorder and are often prescribed lithium (Breggin, 2009), *why are some schools telling parents their child needs to be on more psychotropic medication at risk of expulsion or placement in special education?*

- When "polymedication" is not approved for children by the Federal Drug Administration, or by Health Canada, and is extremely dangerous for children (Baughman, 2009), *why do education and health professionals participate in this practice that is highly unethical, unprofessional and ultimately could kill children?*

- When there is no evidence that use of restraints or locking children in "safe rooms" improves behavior in the long term, and may actually be harmful to children (PENT Forum 2008), *why are schools increasing their use?*

The Dangers of Medicating Children

By simply reducing technology use and increasing outdoor play, schools can improve child attention, behavior and ability to learn. Why then are the education and health professionals increasingly turning to mental heath diagnosis and use of dangerous psychotropic medication, seclusion and restraints to manage child behavior? Is it because it's easy and more cost effective than therapy? One known contributing factor is that in the United States, pharmaceutical companies are allowed to market their drugs to parents and teachers. Everyone has seen stimulant advertisements showing the cute little child who is happily doing their homework? I'd like a child like that, wouldn't you? Misinformation provided to the medical community by fraudulent researchers who were paid by the pharmaceutical industry to "ghost write" research results is more common than we care to believe (New York Times, 2008). Or maybe it was just that prescribing medication became common place and habitual, and health and education professionals have simply forgotten that there are other more safe methods to deal with child behavior.

I recently attended the *International Center for the Study of Psychiatry and Psychology (ICSPP)* conference held in New York in October 2009 titled "Difficult Children and Their Families – Alternatives to Medication" which raised a number of interesting questions about the increasing role the medical profession now plays in the education system. As a medically trained occupational therapist working in the school system for over a decade, I observed first hand the increasing propensity to diagnose and medicate young children. While initially this increasing diagnostic trend seemed to serve the need of the child, as I was able to provide one to one treatment. Soon though, my caseload began to swell, allowing only a consultation service model. I became a "cog" in the ever growing "wheel" of diagnostic categorization for the purpose of much needed educational funding to try to manage children with difficult behaviors.

One disastrous side effect of this "labeling" process was that the health and education professionals somehow became convinced that these children were actually "sick", and had a disease or a chemical imbalance that could only be "fixed" with drugs. What was often a child discipline or behavioral problem, now became a medical condition best managed by use of physical or chemical "restraints". With more and more children being diagnosed, the education system needed more specialist referrals, therapists, special educators, learning assistance personal, and specialized equipment. When the *educational lens* for viewing childhood problems switched to a *medical lens*, the stage was set for how this problem would be interpreted and treated. Diagnosis and medication of children quickly became the norm.

When analyzing trends, it's often informative to use a *global lens* to gain an accurate perspective. Child mental and physical diagnoses, as well as prescriptions for a variety of medications, have sky rocketed in the past decade (Zito, 2002). Does North America really have an epidemic of "sick" children, or might there be another explanation? One proposed theory receiving increasing publicity is that illegal practices of the pharmaceutical industry have misinformed the medical establishment regarding medication efficacy and safety. This has resulted in prolific sales of medication that instead of "curing" child behavior, are quite literally making children permanently mentally and physically disabled, thus ensuring life long use of psychotropic medication.

"It's really the medication side effects that are causing the surge in mental illness, not the other way around," states Dr. Fred Baughman, neurologist and presenter at the ICSPP conference. Dr. Baughman went on to report "Medication is causing irreversible mental illness in many children, and is increasingly being prescribed for behaviors that have no known physical cause." Dr. Baughman presented his correspondence with *Health Canada* and the *Federal Drug Administration* which showed these two regulatory organizations concurred on the following statement "For mental and psychiatric disorders in general, including depression, anxiety, schizophrenia and adhd, there are no confirmatory gross, microscopic or clinical abnormalities that have been validated for objective physical diagnosis. Rather, diagnoses of possible mental conditions are described strictly in terms of patterns of symptoms that tend to cluster together; the symptoms can be observed by the clinician or reported by the patient or family members." When North American drug regulatory agencies concur that mental/psychiatric disorders are not "physical" in origin, but are rather "observed patterns of symptoms", why do the health and education professionals insist on pursuing diagnosis and medication of what could simply be termed "child behavior?"

Dr. Joe Joseph, PhD psychologist and author of *The Gene Illusion* reports there are no known genes for any mental illness (although researchers continue to look), and that previous genetic research is actually based on flawed twin studies which have poor validity and have never been replicated. How many parents are wrongly told by well meaning health and education professionals that their child's behavior is "genetic" in origin and requires medication? If lawyers in the US are successfully litigating against the pharmaceutical industry for fraudulent advertising and withholding negative research findings, how long before the health and education professionals are implicated as well in this rapidly escalating fiasco? Dr. Peter Breggin, author and child psychiatrist states that drugging children makes them "apathetic" and able to sustain attention for long periods on mundane tasks, both traits which continue to be wrongfully interpreted by the health and education establishments as "improvement".

So how can the education and health care systems reverse this maelstrom of professionals convinced that children are "sick" or "learning disabled", and need to be diagnosed and medicated? First and foremost Canadian Health and Education Governments need to step up to the plate to work with child health researchers to develop policies that protect Canadian children. Prohibiting use of psychotropic medications, seclusion rooms and restraints in school settings, would challenge the health and education professionals to adopt more humane methods of managing child behavior. Implementing minimum standards for recess and access to playground structures would optimize socialization and physical development. In the meantime, health and education professionals in the school setting can recommend proven effective alternatives to medication (daily access to "green space", treadmills or stationary bikes for exercise), prohibit personal entertainment technology use, and divert funds from computer upgrades into building "sensational" playgrounds and supervision staff for organized sports. These intervention concepts will be discussed further in Section III.

Chapter 6

Social Communication, Aggression and Isolation

A Father's Devastating Statements Following the Online Posting of a Gang Rape of His 16 Year Old Daughter

We are certainly going after what can be sent, but there's stuff in personal devices that you're never going to be able to stop.

For us, this may just go on and on. To call it a parent's worst nightmare is an understatement...and we're living it.

We are really dealing with a different level of youth and education. The old days are gone. It's out of control. You don't know what to do. You feel helpless.

Excerpt from the Globe and Mail, September 18, 2010

Whether we like it or not, most parents will admit that technology is changing their children, and their children may not be turning into the type of children they want. Unable to socialize without a device, aggressive and violent, utterly lacking in empathy, and spending large amounts of time alone, the new age child is truly a different breed of human. The ability of the 21st century child to socialize with both adults and peers is deteriorating at a rapid pace. Sally Ward, a professor of speech and language pathology reported in her 2004 book "Baby Talk", that one in five toddlers demonstrate speech and language delays. Dimitri Christakis, a pediatric researcher at *Children's Hospital and Regional Medical Center* in Seattle, reports that children learn language skills largely from verbal interactions with their parents. In his recent 2009 study, he placed digital recorders on both parents and children in their homes, Dr. Christakis found that adults typically utter 941 words per hour, yet these adult words are almost completely eliminated when television is audible to the child. Dr. Christakis found that each hour of audible television was associated with significant reductions in child vocalizations, vocalization duration, and conversational turns (when conversation switches from one speaker to the other). On average, each additional hour of television exposure was also associated with a decrease of 770 words the child heard from an adult during the recording session.

With over 50 percent of American households now reporting having the television on continuously, even when no one is watching, researchers interpret these findings have grave implications for language acquisition and early brain development (Christakis, 2009). Parents have stopped talking to their children, impacting not only on their development of speech, but also their ability to socialize with others. My observations during a recent pilot project implemented in a school-based setting in British Columbia, showed one in five kindergarten children demonstrated unintelligible speech and consequent difficulty communicating with teachers and peers. Communication difficulties in the early years have significant impact on not only a child's socialization ability, but also on their ability to be successful in school and eventual work environments. I have observed in home, school and clinic settings that children who have communication impairments have immense frustration as they struggle to get their needs met. Loss of social communication may be one of the most detrimental effects of technology on child development.

The following information profiles the direct impact technology is having on children's social well being, and covers the following areas: empathy, aggression, cyberbullying and sexting, and identity formation.

Empathy

I was recently asked by a friend and colleague Elsje deBoer, whether technology use interfered with the development of interpersonal skills in children, in particular, the way in which they act and react to others in the areas of civility and empathy. This colleague was concerned that parents might be misled by recent research showing that while video games might improve child *problem solving* skill, this skill may come at the price of increased aggression, often in the form of bullying. Civility is defined as "politeness" and valuing the esteem of another. Empathy is defined as understanding and being able to share the feelings of another. Bullying is defined as intent to hurt or intimidate another, and often involves aggression or violent actions. I would like to propose that child technology use might be a limiting factor in the development of civility and empathy in children.

Our Inner Ape by Frans de Waal states "Empathy stems from the recognition and imitation of facial expression, body language and tone of voice". As the development of civility and empathy both require personal interactions with others, one might wonder how children can value or care for one another if they don't interact with them. Children who engage in excessive screen time will have difficulty developing civility and empathy, as they are limited in achieving adequate personal interaction with their peers. Use of the aforementioned *Technology Guidelines* would offer additional information regarding what type of technology, how often is it used, how long is it used, how violent is it, how old is the child, and is the child using this type of technology in isolation or with friends. One might think that children playing videogames together are interacting personally, yet in recent film footage shot by Robbie Cooper of children playing videogames (see robbiecooper.org *Simulations - Immersions*) this does not appear to be the case. Whether there are other children in the room or not, playing video games is ultimately an activity of isolation, thus limiting development of civility and empathy.

A 2010 University of Michigan study shows today's college students are 40-percent less empathetic than those of the 1980s and 1990s determined by an analysis of the past 30 years of students who participated in the *Davis Interpersonal Reactivity Index*. This index looked at empathic concern, emotional response to the distress of others, and "perspective-taking" or the ability to imagine another person's perspective. This study cites the influx of callous reality television shows and the growth of social networking and texting as causal factors for the decline in empathy in today's young people (Globe and Mail, 2010). Recent incidents of growing child aggression against other children and school staff members have been reported in the press to have doubled in the Vancouver School District in the past three years (Vancouver Sun, 2010). School management difficulties with increasing numbers of aggressive children, is resulting in the rising use of physical and chemical restraints, as well as a rising use of seclusion rooms (Gaskin, 2007; Vancouver Sun 2010; Muralidharan, 2009). Civility and empathy may well be traits of the past.

Seclusion Rooms

Isolating a child who exhibits unmanageable behavior, and who also is likely to have a failed primary attachment with their primary parent(s), seems counterintuitive to say the least. When a child really needs a hug, do we want to lock them in a room, devoid of any human interaction or connection? Who are we protecting? While these procedures may resolve the immediate issue of a violent child, the long term benefits are few, and studies show the use of seclusion rooms may cause irreversible harm and even death (PENT Forum, 2008). Schools may want to consider potential legal implications of locking children in seclusion rooms, and ensure prevention initiatives have been employed and alternatives trialed before they proceed with this dangerous practice.

Aggression

An "aggressive act" is defined in the research literature as one of "intentional harm". Historically, aggression has played a societal role for humankind, and has even been documented as an innate trait found in animals. What is a stark contrast between today's world and the worlds of generations past, is that entertainment technology has literally *immersed* us in violence. 95% of video games, 75% of television shows and 60% of cartoons contain violent acts (Huesmann, 2007). While these statistics may seem hard to believe, there are literally millions of options for viewing violent media content, as practically every television show is now accessible on the internet, by everyone, no matter what their age.

There is an overwhelming body of evidence that links violent media content to increased aggression in children. In *Violent Video Game Effects on Children and Adolescents: Theory, Research and Public Policy*, authors Craig Anderson, Douglas Gentile, and Katherine Buckley report "There is unequivocal evidence that media violence increases the likelihood of aggressive and violent behavior in both immediate and long term contexts." This book documents empirical research on the effects of violent video games, and explores public policy options for controlling their distribution. Authors report that "violence sells", and accurately profile concerns regarding regulating an industry that is clearly driven by monetarily interests, without consideration for the outcomes of product use. At what point do the producers of violent media content (film, video games, television, and internet) accept responsibility for the fruits of their labors? At what point should government and researchers step in and begin to regulate and legislate media violence?

Dr. David Birkham from the *Boston Children's Hospital Center for Media Research* reports that the higher the exposure and intensity of media violence, the more likely the child is to develop bullying behavior, and even become incarcerated upon adulthood (online webinar, 2009). A 2008 study by Craig A. Anderson with Iowa State University's *Center for the Study of Violence* showed video game use was causally linked to increased school fighting, as well as increased identification by a teacher or peer as being aggressive. The study goes on to report that "In the short-term, media violence increases aggression by priming aggressive thoughts and decision processes, increasing physiological arousal, and triggering a tendency to imitate observed behaviors. In the long-term, repeated exposure can produce lasting increases in aggressive thought patterns and aggression-supporting beliefs about social behavior, and can reduce individuals normal negative emotional responses to violence." Based on these research results, it does appear that violent media turns some children into bullies, thus necessitating an accompanying technology reduction component in all bullying prevention and treatment programs.

The *Committee on Public Education* with the American Academies of Pediatrics, Physicians, Psychiatrists, and Psychologists report the following character traits are associated with viewing violent media content:

- Increased physiological arousal
- Chronic release of cortisol (adrenalin)
- Desensitization
- Increased aggressive thought patterns
- Hostile personalities
- Pro-violent attitudes
- Increased anti-social and aggressive behavior
- Increased verbal and physical abuse

- Viewing the world as violent and mean
- Fear of being harmed
- Night terrors and nightmares
- Desire to see more violence in entertainment and real life
- Viewing violence as an acceptable way to resolve conflict

Today's technology addicted child is hardwiring his or her brain for violent high-speed and fast-paced action, resulting in an unprecedented rise in child aggression, violence and crime (Anderson, 2007; Anderson, 2006; Anderson, 2008; Murray, 2006; Buchanan, 2002). In the United States, the Academies of Physicians, Pediatricians, Psychologists, and Psychiatrists have joined with the American Medical Association to classify media violence as a "public health risk" due to its impact on child aggression, with eventual plans to legislate the regulation of media violence allowed for viewing by children (Huesmann, 2007). As discussed previously, researchers report that neural pathway formation in children who overuse technology is "short-circuiting" the frontal cortex, *permanently* altering the way children think and behave (Small, 2008). As brain development involves the "pruning" of neurons that are not in use, the natural product of technology overuse by children is the loss of neurons that project to the frontal cortex. The frontal cortex controls executive functioning and "impulse control". The over use of entertainment technologies that contain violent content, and the "pruning" of neurons that project to the frontal cortex, may in fact be creating a generation of children who will not be literate and who will be impulsive - a deadly combination for the perpetration of violence.

The definition of "impulse" is a compulsion that one cannot control. The most dangerous and potentially harmful impulse is that of aggression and violence, which kills hundreds of children in North America every year. Another impulse is the engagement in addictive behaviors. Combine a person who is unable to control violent outbursts, with drugs and alcohol, and we have potentially significant problems coming our way, in fact, they are already here. In 2008 a 27 year old man from Philadelphia was playing on his Xbox when his 17-month-old daughter pulled on some cords and tipped the Xbox to the ground, breaking it. The father reportedly became so enraged that he struck his daughter with such force, and so many times, that it cracked her skull causing death (CBS News, 2008). While the father was remorseful following his daughter's death, if the same situation presented itself, would he react in the same way? Very likely. Researchers indicate that children who overuse video games, after they were restricted from all technology use for a period of one year, still had not re-formed neuronal tracks to their frontal lobes (Murray, 2006). This research documents a frightening fact: once impulse control is gone from human ability, it may never come back.

Cyberbullying and Sexting

When parents don't place restrictions on technology use, or train their young ones in appropriate use of technologies, these parents will have technology use management problems, both in homes and schools. Two of these problem areas are cyberbullying and sexting.

The term "cyberbullying" is so new that my spell check still identifies it as misspelled, but is so pervasive that studies now show over twenty-five percent of elementary-aged school children have been cyberbullied, meaning they have been bullied online (Ybarra, 2007). Even though cyberbullying occurs online and generally is enacted while children are at home, the fear and violence is usually enacted on the school grounds, creating an interesting dilemma for school staff, as how can they control something that happens online in homes? Due to the profound fear these children who suffer from cyberbullying experience, children who have been cyberbullied have an increased risk of carrying a weapon to school by eight times (Kowalski, 2007; Ybarra, 2007). This fact in and of itself should strike fear in the hearts of every parent, and should be incentive enough to restrict at least their own child's technology use.

Young children who "sextext" (e-mail nude photos using cell phones) are presently being arrested for distribution of child pornography (Garfinkle, 2008). Really? Where is the role of the parents and teachers in the education of children regarding safe use of technology? Would we put guns or drugs in the hands of young children? Certainly not – yet we hand them cell phones, digital cameras, and access to the internet. Without so much as a thought as to what these children will do with these devices, we just send them off to school with lunches, a warm coat and cell phones that could get them arrested if improperly used. These "crimes of technology" indicate that many children do not have the maturity or the parental guidance to use technology in a safe and responsible manner.

Civility and empathy training are integral components for cyberbullying and sexting education, prevention and treatment programs. Civility and empathy training not only improve the psychological well being of the individual, but also are important for development of conflict resolution with others. Personal interaction time with others is necessary in order to resolve conflict, and is therefore another justification for initiating technology awareness and reduction programs in school-based settings. When considering existing levels of global and domestic violence, imagine a world where individuals are unable to resolve conflict. Safety would be a rarity, and schools, homes and communities would need to become heavily guarded and patrolled. Add the current state of world conflict to the ramifications of a future generation of violent videogame addicts, and we have a very scary situation indeed.

Identity Formation

The impact of technology overuse on the formation of self identity is an integral component to the formation of a child's ability to form social relationships with others. As children immerse themselves deeper into the solitary world of the *virtual realm*, their ability to determine who they are, separate from the television or video game character, becomes increasingly difficult. Children younger than the age of eight years have difficulty distinguishing the difference between games or play that is "fantasy" in origin, and games or play that is grounded in reality (Buchanan, 2002). With increasing exposure to violent media content at a younger and younger age, erosion of the already fragile development of self identity, human relatedness and formation of empathy can be expected. Daniel Petric, an adolescent from Ohio who shot and killed his mother and disabled his father after they confiscated his Halo 3 video game, told the judge upon being sentenced, "I didn't know that it (the gun) was real. I thought that they (his parents) would come back to life." (News.com.au, 2009).

A 2008 comprehensive study by researchers from the *National Institute of Health* and Yale University analyzed 173 research efforts on the impact of technology on children and found that 80% showed a link between media hours or content with negative health outcomes such as obesity, tobacco use, sexual behavior, drug and alcohol use, low academic achievement and incidence of adhd. Research co-author Cary P. Gross states "We need to realize that children are sponges, learning from their environment" and that "Children pick up character traits and behaviors from what they watch and hear." I frequently tell parents that a child's brain is like a camera, recording everything they see, so they better be careful what their child watches, because it will be with them forever.

A premise in occupational therapy is that "we are what we do", and to be physically and mentally healthy, we need to engage in "meaningful" activity. If the only activity a child engages in or finds meaningful is technology, then this is who they will become. A robotic automaton who is completely unable to connect with other human beings, and who spends endless hours engaged with – you got it – a device. I was asked to assess the motor and sensory skills, as well as behavior of a 4 year old boy who had been "expelled" from his daycare due to aggression. What struck me as odd as soon as I walked through the door, was that this child was glued, and I mean *glued* to the television. He was watching a cartoon, and when I asked the parent to turn it off, she said that he would have a tantrum as this was one of his favorite shows. I stated that I needed to observe his "range" of behaviors, which I did, when the television was turned off. This child "became" one of the characters he was watching in on the television, including bringing with him an array of weapons. As I thought it wise to include myself in his fantasy until we had established a "rapport", I carried on being his opponent, play fighting with him with his imaginary weapons. When I said "Okay, that's enough, my real name is Cris, what's your name?", this child continued on being the television character, for the rest of the two hour session. His Mom stated that her son never responds to his name, only to specific characters from television or video games. While this was "cute" when he was 2 and 3 years of age, his Mom readily stated that she was somewhat worried, and even a little scared, as her son always chose to be a character with a fair degree of aggression.

Needless to say, we focused on establishing a connection between Mom and child, using attachment building techniques discussed in Section III, and this child slowly started the long journey toward relating not only to his mother, but to himself. Connection to technology is disconnecting children, from themselves, others and nature. Allowing a child to "disconnect" from all that is human and "real" will relegate them to a life full of sadness and despair. I implore all parents reading this book, to put it down and go hug your child. Read to them, play with them, ask them how their day was, and listen to what they have to say. All parents have to do is listen to their child's story, feel their pain. Children miss their parents more than they can say, and only choose technology because parents aren't there for them. This may be the hardest thing you as a parent will ever do, but your child needs you, and without you, they will perish.

It's October and Halloween time. My daughter has always considered Halloween to be a serious occasion. I think she views Halloween as a time to indulge her "alter" ego and become whoever she was "meant to be". Grade 8 she was a chimney sweep, grade 9 Edward Scissorhands, grade 10 a Twister Board, and this year Uma Thurman in the movie Kill Bill.

My daughter makes her own costumes, and generally does a pretty decent job, but this year she went all out. Her Auntie Val bought her yards of bright yellow "pleather" and she made skin tight pants and jacket, complete with Harley and racing emblems, and of course a sword. She looked great.

But this year she came home from school sad and dejected because "No one wants to dress up anymore!" When she started high school, she said "everyone" dressed up, and now it's only about half the school that makes an effort. She also said the costumes weren't nearly as good as they used to be back when she was in grade 8.

It seems ironic doesn't it, that the more we immerse ourselves in a virtual world, the less imagination and creativity we have to live in the real world.

Imagination is a sad thing to loose.

Cris Rowan, Author, 2010

Chapter 7

Academic Performance

Concerns Regarding Education Technology

There has been a movement in education toward increased reliance on technology. Unfortunately, often times technology has been blindly adopted without the important study of its impact on child development. Educators have been so busy adapting to new ways of instruction, that change so rapidly, that we have been flying by the seat of our pants and are left in a quandary as to why. Since technology is supposed to be a panacea, we are having to deal with more and more problems with behavior and learning in our classrooms.

Lisa Ford, High School Math Teacher, British Columbia

There likely isn't a parent, teacher or therapist out there who doesn't think technology is educational. There are technology programs that can teach infants to read, toddlers to text message and do math, and of course once they get into school, can teach elementary-aged children to do just about anything. There are downsides to this line of thinking, as technology can no more prepare children for the future than could a robot. Children need movement, touch and human connection to grow up healthy and succeed in this world, and none of that comes in an electrical device. It would be so easy (and cost effective) if we could just hand our children a device and it would do everything for us. Teach them, raise them, entertain them, and make sure they were loved and safe and happy. While technology can do many things, it also *can't* do these things. We need to determine *who, what, when, where, why* and *how* technology can assist a child's learning quickly, before we make mistakes that will be impossible to reverse.

The *National Center for Education Statistics in 2005* reported that early exposure to printed text through the reading of books and learning to print is the largest predictor of literacy. Only 60% of high school graduates ever achieve the literacy skills employers seek. Despite this knowledge, many schools are foregoing printed textbooks and reducing educator time spent teaching children to print, in favor of using computers as teaching tools for young children. Without any knowledge regarding the possible differences between screen reading and book reading, whole school districts, without any research evidence to support this decision, are rapidly moving toward the use of computers as "virtual teachers" for elementary aged children. An article in a technology journal *Fast Company* in April, 2010 referenced teachers as mere "moderators" in the learning process, and intimated that many children will soon be able to do their "work" from home. Referred to as the "$100 curriculum in a box" by educational technology companies, devices such as TeacherMates and XO's are expected in the near future to actually replace teachers.

While a few children may survive this transition from real to virtual, the majority will not. Many children require a more "hands on" approach to learning that involves a human element, and these type of children will not do well learning from a device. This line of thinking by educators that technology can teach every child everything they need to succeed in their future, is short sighted and likely to result in profound ramifications for our children. Literacy, socialization with peers, empathy, and the ability to print, are being tossed aside for what is thought to be "progressive" teaching and learning. "Throwing the baby out with the bathwater" mentality by the education system is leading us down a perilous road, and we have no idea where it will take us. Short term solutions to the long standing problem of attaining literacy are never a good idea, and are likely to cause the demise of the whole educational framework as we once knew it. How can anyone state that computers should become universal learning tools, when there has not been one valid long term study to support this unfounded belief. Researchers are limited in their ability to perform long term studies, because technology is evolving faster than they can design, implement, analyze and publish their research. Without long term, valid and reproducible studies, the education system is "flying by the seat of their pants" so to speak, and operating with one dimensional "blinders".

The following information profiles the direct impact technology is having on children's *academic performance*, and covers the following areas: illiteracy; inattention and impulsivity, educational technology; and the dangers of school-based technology.

Illiteracy

In school settings I have witnessed an increased practice of educators to provide children who have printing, reading or learning difficulties, a laptop, with minimal knowledge regarding whether or not this device can actually improve their literacy. Literacy is defined as competency in handwriting, reading, numerical and communication skill, and is a foundation for the successful achievement of academic and social competence (Shanahan, 2007). Studies from the *United Kingdom Literacy Association* indicate that we have limited knowledge about the comparative aspects of screen reading vs. book reading, and suggest that they are two totally different ways of learning, and consequently require different instructional methods. This study pointed to the fact that computers don't teach students how to critically analyze internet information, and the speed with which it is presented prohibits adequate processing time for retention and application. Preliminary research studies indicate that screen reading is not as effective as book reading in number of key aspects, and raises caution for switching over to screen reading as a universal teaching tool (Mangan, 2008). Current research reports poorer academic performance for screen reading compared to book reading in the following areas:

- Attention: clicking and scrolling disrupt attention and disturb mental appreciation
- Comprehension: reader lacks both completeness and constituent parts
- Memory: change in physical surroundings has a negative effect on memory
- Learning: doesn't allow required time and mental exertion
- Meaning: isn't a physical dimension, loss of totality

One thing computers will never be able to do is to teach children how to print, yet teachers everywhere have pretty much quit printing instruction, even in the primary grades of kindergarten to grade three. Ester Goldberg and Marvin Simner, professors with University of Alberta reported as early as 1999 the importance of teaching children to print as a precursor to reading and speech fluency, and found that poor handwriting skill is related to language disorders. 20 years ago in Canada, printing used to be a curriculum based subject, with standards for instruction and evaluation methods, and instruction time averaged one hour per day in the primary grades. Now, a 2008 study by Steven Graham found that primary teachers spend an inadequate 13 minutes per day teaching handwriting skills, even though the majority of a child's *graded output* requires written (not computer) performance. Teachers seem to be under the illusion that technology will solve every child's problems, but they forgot that the majority of student examination requires students to print.

Children who don't know the mechanics of printing never develop what is termed by occupational therapists as a "motor plan" for automatic, subconscious letter and number production. These struggling printers produce poor quality and quantity of print, as each time the pencil hits the paper the child has to think about where to start, which way to go, and when to stop when making their letters or numbers. Not having achieved automatic printing in the primary years, impacts a child's eventual academic performance in every subject, as slow printers have difficulty with spelling, sentence production, short answers (socials and science), and math. Children who are slow printers have been observed to become easily frustrated and upset, and may proceed toward development of significant behavior issues, as they are asked numerous times a day to do something they were never taught how to do. Not knowing the mechanics of printing also significantly impacts on a child's ability to read and speak, as the motor planning required for automatic letter production when printing "maps" the sensorimotor cortex for eventual visual letter recognition for reading, and even for word finding in oral sentence production (Goldberg, 1999; Tomblin, 2006). The movement of the education system toward virtual learning through use of computers has limited research and no long term studies to support this wide spread initiative. This ill informed decision may result in a whole generation of children lost to illiteracy. Will this matter, will children need literacy in the future, or will internet surfing suffice?

I've been asked on numerous occasions to teach printing to high school students who are required to print legibly for a job placement who still struggle with written output. Even in the age of computers, job entry frequently requires printing skill, which many of our high school graduates fail to achieve. Why is this? Children cannot learn to print through osmosis, although many teachers seem to think they can. Children require strategy based instruction using consistent methods for instruction and evaluation. This type of teaching no longer exists in our *progressive* technology driven educational environments, and as a result, illiteracy rates continue to climb. Can computers replace the need for job entry literacy? While we don't know the answers to these questions now, as there is limited research in the area of computer literacy, we'll sadly soon find out.

Inattention and Impulsivity

Numerous studies indicate technology overuse by children is causally related to attention difficulties and poor academic achievement (Christakis, 2007; Hancox, 2005; Swing, 2010). Dr. Dimitri Christakis with the University of Washington found in a 2004 study that each hour of television watched daily between the ages of 0 and 7 years of age, equated to a 10% increase in attention problems by age 7 years. So, children who use 7.5 hours per day of technology reasonably could have a 75% higher incidence of attention problems. Every educator would be wise to carefully consider the implications of this study when they are recommending a child use technology as part of their learning curriculum. Children who are unable to pay attention, are unable to learn. Well, maybe they can learn something they are interested in, like how to navigate an underground tunnel to get to their opponent's lair in a video game. This generally is not the type of information we want our children to learn at school, and likely not the type of skills they need for job entry. Nearly every child I talk to about what they are going to do for work once they graduate, tell me "Design video games!" To learn information such as social studies, science or math, children are required to slow their brains down, and pay attention to follow the instruction from the teacher.

Many teachers and education administrators erroneously believe that computers will teach all of these subjects, and in a fun and entertaining manner. While there may actually be education programs that profess to do this, the outcomes have not likely been measured, and these programs are therefore largely untested. Concern arises when we consider previously presented research regarding the "pruning" of neuronal tracks to the frontal lobes known for impulsivity control, necessary for attention and learning (Small, 2008, Murray, 2006). Will long term use of fast paced educational technology result in the "pruning" of the brain, effectively eliminating the educational aspects altogether? Only quality, long term research will give us these answers.

Educational Technology

Just as with pharmaceutical companies, educational technology production companies should be required to produce outcome studies that meet rigorous criteria for acceptance into a school-based curriculum. The studies should be performed by an independent firm with no financial ties to the outcomes, and demonstrate reliable and replicated results. These studies should be performed on a wide range of student abilities, and on students who both *under* and *over* use technology. Long term studies of educational technologies should be required prior to wide scale use. Who knows what the long term results will be for use of a computer program for teaching reading in the primary grades.

There is a new movement in the education industry to pattern educational programs after video games. While the premise is understandable, children do demonstrate excellent attention to video games, the end result may be that we have created more problems than we've solved. For instance, presenting information in a fast and entertaining manner may not result in long term retention for eventual application of this information. How many of us sit down and look something up on Google, only to forget whatever the information was once we stand up? While the information might be presented in an appeasing manner, the process of "surfing" may be counterintuitive to saving this information in long term, retrievable memory. As the information was presented rapidly, we unfortunately never engaged our frontal lobes to *process* the information, and so forgot it as soon as the screen shifted to a new topic. The 21st century is renown for "breath" without "depth", which is not conducive to long term memory and learning.

Dr. Gary Small reports in his book *iBrain* that "While the brains of today's children are wiring up for rapid fire cyber searches, the neural circuits that control the more traditional learning methods are neglected and gradually diminish". Dr. Samll discusses another study by Professor Akio Mori with Tokyo Nihon University found that the use of video games actually *suppress* frontal lobe activity thus gravely limiting attention ability, and that chronic players who play greater that 2 hours per day actually develop "video game brain", a syndrome that essentially turns off the frontal lobes, even when kids are not playing video games. Video game brain in a classroom setting simply does not allow the level of attention required for learning. Dr. Small proposes "Are we rearing a new generation with underdeveloped frontal lobes – a group of young people unable to learn, remember, feel, or control their impulses? Or will they develop new advanced skills that will poise them for extraordinary achievements?" We don't know. Managing technology use in home and school settings, as well as increasing children's access to outdoor playgrounds and activities, appears to be a much more cost effective and healthy alternative to use of educational technology.

When physical exercise has been shown to significantly reduce impulsivity and improve attention (Ratey, 2008), and access to "green space" restores attention and significantly reduces adhd (Faber-Taylor, 2001; Kuo, 2004), current practices by the health and education professionals to place them in front of computers, and then medicate children with attention difficulties, simply does not make sense.

The Dangers of School Technology – What We Don't Know

Several scientists from around the world testified about the dangers of microwave transmissions during parliamentary hearings into cellular telephones in the spring of 2010 (CBC News, 2010). Both cell phones and Wi-Fi (wireless internet) utilize microwave radiation. Critics point out that exposure to radiation from Wi-Fi is often for hours at a time, not minutes as it is with cell phones. These scientists have brought much needed attention to what could become a significant problem in school settings, the prevalent use of wireless internet. "Symptoms referred to as microwave syndrome, like headaches, sleep disturbances, fatigue, etc., among people residing around base station antennas can possibly be explained by cellular stress induction on brain cells or even cell death," testified Dimitri Panagopoulos, a biophysicist from the University of Athens. Prof. Olle Johansson of the *Royal Institute of Technology* in Sweden warned the committee that Canada and other countries need to update their guidelines for exposure to microwave radiation. "It's obvious that your safety code is completely out of date and obsolete and that goes for any form of international or national standard body throughout the world," testified Johansson.

We really just don't know what is down the "educational pipe" in the area of technology, do we? Are we going to find that all these devices emit harmful radiation, or will we find out we were worried about nothing? Likely, the answers will fall somewhere in between. Likely we will find out that these devices are harmful to young children, but as their brains develop, will affect them less so. Likely we will find out that if we keep within limits set by our medical and research communities, our children will be okay. But many schools are not even keeping within these guidelines now. Young children are often using greater than the 1-2 hours per day recommended by the experts *at school*, and then use an average of 7.5 hours per day far more when they get home. What if I'm wrong? What if these devices are *extremely* harmful to everyone's physical, mental, social and productive health, what then?

Acting with caution now will certainly not harm anyone, and could stand to benefit everyone. The above noted research should raise alarm and is a call to action for parents, teachers and health professionals. While the implications of this research are far reaching and nothing short of profound, more research needs to be generated to validate and replicate these findings in order to provide informed guidelines for technology use restrictions. In the meanwhile, to sit and do nothing will most likely prove harmful to children. When in doubt, erring on the side of caution is a wise guideline to follow. But how cautious should we be, and should we be more cautious with younger children, than adolescents those of high school age?

Technology is like a fast moving train that has left the station and is charging full steam ahead, without adequate research regarding the long term effects on child physical, mental, social and academic performance. No one seems to have noticed that children are falling off this fast paced technology train, at a rapid rate. Maybe it's time to bring the train back to the station, and design proper outcome based research to evaluate both the short and long term effects of technology overuse on children. Dramatic changes to existing health and education theory and techniques without adequate supporting research, may result in unfavorable outcomes. I'm now ending my section profiling the research regarding the *direct* or causal effects of technology on children, and will move onto talking about *indirect* or secondary effects.

Indirect Effects - Impact of Technology in Homes, Schools and Communities

Thoughts on Conscious Awareness

It is imperative that we nurture the seeds we have planted, Our Children.

To recognize and truly understand that in this very moment, our children are creating the world in which they live in, now and after we are gone.

The responsibility lies within each and every one of us to "Wake Up". There are many people that recognize this and are helping in a conscious way.

It is the babies, toddlers, children, tweens, and teens that need to know they are born in a special time, when technology and consciousness are being integrated.

Our future generation has a choice to realize they are alive, and to "Live Life" and develop their special gifts and talents so that they can use technology in a healthy and balanced way.

The way is through Conscious Awareness.

Technology is no substitute for life. We cannot sustain life or our planet in a VIRTUAL REALITY.

Cheryl Metz, Dancer, Muse and Visionary, British Columbia

The impact of 21st century technology on our children has been most pronounced in our homes and schools, yet we rarely allow ourselves the time to think about or process these changes. We're just too busy! Bringing conscious awareness to the world around us is imperative, if we are ever able to integrate technology into our lives in a responsible and enlightened way.

The next two chapters will profile the *indirect* or secondary changes to our family and school structures that have seen incredible change from technology. We often don't allow ourselves the opportunity to contemplate how different our lives have become over the past decade, and whether these changes have enhanced our family and school lives, or made us more stressed and unhappy. Sometimes it's a good thing to reflect on the past. Was life simpler, less complex and confusing? Were we *more* or *less* connected to your family and students?

I'm certainly not suggesting we turn back the clock, but taking this time to reflect on the ways of the past, could help everyone figure out what is working for them right now with reference to technology, and what isn't. Technology isn't the answer to every problem, and sometimes technology is the *cause* of our problems. Sorting through these issues takes some time. Close your eyes, take three deep breaths, and read on.

Remember back when we were children? We used to run, jump and play all day, riding bikes, building forts and rough housing in an imaginary world of games we made up all on our own? Playground swings and slides were high and long, giving us a rush of stomach "butterflies", with fast merry-go-rounds and challenging jungle gyms. We rode our bikes or walked to school, and often stayed after school for an organized group or sport activity. On the way home we might stop at a store and get some candy, or play in a park or local wooded area. We moved all the time, and through play, experienced essential touch and connection with other human beings, all crucial factors for normal child development. Play was highly creative and required minimal manufactured toys or specialized equipment, as everything was either imaginary or found in nature. A stick, branch or rock could become a whole city of make believe creatures, with moss for hair and a leaf for a dress. I remember spending hours with my friends jumping off the roof of an abandoned house, hanging onto a tree branch and bouncing and up and down, laughing the whole time. My parents now say they never worried about us kids, where we were or whether we were getting kidnapped or bullied. They said they knew we were somewhere between school and home, playing, like kids should.

As a child and young adult, our family spent most summers at "the cabin" on a lake in Oregon, where we had many adventures, and many "misadventures". We camped, rowed leaky rowboats, jumped off 30' cliffs (into the water), and rode a rubber raft with no floor down river rapids. I remember one time our "raft" flipped and I got stuck underneath. When we reached my Dad who was waiting at the causeway, I was crying and spurting water, with my two brothers telling me to "quit acting like a girl". My Dad quietly packed us back into the car and drove us back up river to do it all over again, saying he was worried that if I didn't get back on that river right away, I might never go down again. We did that ride, and I have to say, there isn't much that scared me as I was growing up, or even in my adult life today.

When we finally got home from all our adventures, us kids would talk with our parents about what happened that day, generally over the dinner table, and often again before bedtime. While these dinner table discussions went far longer than I would have liked at the time, thinking back now, these family talks were memorable times that formed a large part of who I am today, conversations that helped to form my identity. We had a huge back yard where everyone in the neighborhood would come to play. While we were relegated to our obligatory dinner table conversation, the neighborhood children would have their noses pressed up to the sliding glass door, waiting for our eventual "release" from captivity.

It was a different world back then, a world that seems far away and sometimes very hard to remember. I was telling a "leaky row boat" story recently at one of my workshops for teachers, and my Mom was visiting so she came along and was in the audience. I stopped talking and asked my Mom if she was ever worried about us kids, rowing across the lake in a leaky row boat and jumping off 30 foot cliffs and she responded "Oh no dear, you kids were having so much fun! I had time to myself, and would sew curtains, bake cookies, or paint a wall or two in the cabin. It was actually quite nice to have you out of my hair!"

My family and nature adventures were a huge part of my life as a child. Even now as an adult with children of my own, I continue to pass on my ingrained values in the form of family dinners, kayak adventures, holiday traditions, and parties. Family structures and systems have certainly changed, and I'm not all that sure that the changes are for the good.

Words of Wisdom from a Wife, Mother and Grandmother

Time is one of the most important gifts we have. We need to constantly evaluate our use and possible abuse of this gift. If children spend an inordinate amount of time using technology, it means they are missing out on many of the other helpful building blocks to their development.

Following are just a few of those beneficial building blocks:

Free play time - Unstructured playtime (with little or no adult intervention) brings out a child's creativity, e.g., building a tent under the kitchen table; baking mud pies; tea parties; exploring the neighborhood; meeting new friends and neighbors; tree houses; and hiding places. In the process, very often children go outside, get physical exercise without thinking about it, and learn to "work together" on projects. Those with leadership qualities get a chance to develop them. Those who prefer to follow learn to recognize the importance of their role.

Reading – Probably takes one of the biggest hits from technology. Very often when given the choice of watching TV, playing a video game or reading, children are attracted to the activity requiring the least amount of effort. Their choice of technology limits their growth mentally, and socially. In addition to increasing their proficiency, reading with or to someone can be a growing and bonding experience.

Disposition – Years ago when TV first came out, I observed a big change in the disposition of our 3 children. After an hour of TV the children got quite irritable and "spaced out." We didn't even have the other technologies at that time so TV was my primary concern. I found that if I required them to do something physical, they became more "balanced."

Physical Activity – Also looses out to the attractive passive activity of TV. Some of the video games have addressed that and are somewhat better—just don't inspire much creativity. Going for a walk with someone opens doors to develop communication skills in addition to the physical activity. A good swim or bicycle ride has many benefits.

Keep a good balance!!

Val Schmitt, author's mother and grandmother to five, Oregon.

Chapter 8

Disintegration of the Family

When I was a child growing up, my favorite night was Sunday, when we would gather in front of the television, dinner on metal folding trays, and we would watch Lassie, Flipper and then Disney. I love animals, and in these shows, the animal was always the hero, as they always saved the day. I would go to bed thinking that the world was a safe place to be. I mean after all, we do have Lassie, Flipper and Old Yeller looking out for us, don't we?

Safe – But At What Cost?

For better or worse, today's families are very different from families of the past. Children of today are exposed to a far different visual experience than children of past times, and instead of going to bed feeling happy and safe, many of our children are trying to fall asleep at night feeling scared and anxious. Why? Many parents perceive that the world is "unsafe" and consequently keep their children indoors, away from nature, friends and generally speaking, all things that are natural and human. This "fear" that parents have of the unknown, is largely due to media proliferation of very scary events, such as child abductions or murders by psychopaths. While these events may have happened thousands of miles away, television and internet play these events over and over, instilling fear into every fiber and cell of a parent's body. Children sense their parent's fear even if they are not told about these gruesome events. Children will "feel" a parent's fear, and it will make them scared and anxious.

A study by Burdette in 2005, found that a mother's perceptions of safety determined their children's television viewing time, and that a mother who perceived the world as "unsafe", allowed their children to watch more television. While we should applaud parents efforts to keep their children safe, indoor environments are highly restrictive to the necessary rough and tumble play and imaginative conversations that should happen out in back yards, playgrounds, and in nature with classmates, family and friends. Creating imaginary games and role playing are crucial to the development of an expansive and productive mind. Many parents don't realize that television and video games are akin to "spoon feeding" their children with pre-programmed thoughts and manufactured ideas, limiting a child's ability to produce their own way of thinking. Al Gore in his book *Assault on Reason* implies that the one-way medium of television is "dumbing down" our generation, and removing the two-way option for questions and critical analysis of what is going on around us. Independent thought is imperative in the development of a child's self worth and establishment of their own identity.

The Great Escape

Parents are and always will be the corner stone of a healthy and happy family unit, and parents therefore play an integral role in modeling appropriate behaviors. When today's parent arrives home, after working long, busy days, they are frequently tired and therefore unable to be emotionally available to their children. Exhausted parents come home to phone messages, emails, and neglected dogs and children who really need to go for a walk. Instead of going outdoors and getting "physical", which would give family members the restorative fresh air and exercise they really need, tired parents often find themselves reaching for the remote to escape from the daily pressures of life. The fast pace of today's society is greatly limiting quality time spent in a connected way with family members. While technology offers immediate and instant gratification, it has also left many adults feeling frazzled, mentally exhausted and in need of "down time", so they "veg out" in front of the television.

Studies have found the number one reason adults use technology is to "escape" (Block, 2008). I've pondered this concept endlessly. Why are we living lives in which we feel we need to escape? Escape from what and whom, and escape to where – a place better or more interesting than what we now have? I really don't understand reality television or *Second Life* avatar games, both of which transport the viewer for a time into another world. I was at the dentist recently and everyone, except me, was talking about a contestant on a reality dance show, almost as if he were a sibling, or a child of their own. They seemed to know more about this person than members of their own family, and had definite ideas and passions about why or why not their favorite dancer should win the competition. Why are we more interested in strangers than our own friends and family? Why do we feel we are living a life from which we need to escape to another, why don't we just change the life we are living? Why don't we get out of whatever it is that is so intolerable that it requires "escape", and go somewhere else? With all the advancements made in transportation and communication technologies, why should any of us be living a life in which we feel trapped and unhappy?

Social networking, while designed to improve communication has achieved exactly the opposite. While people think and report they are more "connected", studies reveal that social networking results in people feeling more lonely, less connected, and more anxious than those who use non-technology forms of communication such as the phone or live visits (Khurana, 2009). While the "breadth" is there, and people can communicate with long lost relatives and high school friends, there is apparently little "depth" in these communications, leaving the participant feeling more sad and lonely than they were before (social networking). Communicating for long periods with people they hardly know, as opposed to spending quality time with their close family and friends, may indicate that a person has a personal comfort in, or preference for, isolation. As depression is associated with isolation, this choice of isolation may pose a problem for people and/or their loved ones.

No Time to Talk

Time occupied with technology has gravely impacted on "meaningful" communication between parents and children, which is now reduced to a mere 3.5 minutes per week (Turcotte, 2004), where meaningful communication is defined as something other than "care giving". Gone are the days of lengthy family discussions, playful rough housing and sibling rivalry with youngsters, with endless parental lectures regarding what kids should wear, who they could play with, and how late they could stay outside and play. Gone is the family dining room table, having been slowly replaced by the big screen. Television watching has reduced family conversation to occasional guttural comments about who's doing what on *American Idol*, or who gets voted off *Survivor*. These "conversations" seem to hold more importance and value than homework, a bad report card, or a recent bullying incident or argument with a best friend.

The replacement of the dining room table with television has caused extensive damage to the family unit, as the art of communication has been lost, and family members haven't a clue these days how to have a conversation. An electrical failure resulting from a recent wind storm left my community without power for a period of three very long days. I heard stories that ranged from families feeling frustrated and resorting to frequent arguments, right up to absolute family "meltdowns" of rage, with bouts of crying and despair as they struggled to cope with no television, video games, cell phones or computers. The fact that these families had no heat, refrigeration or lights didn't appear to be of any significance compared to the profound effects of life without technology!

With regard to family conversations, many of us may remember our own dinner time experiences as not being particularly interesting. However, the dining room experience did offer a unique and essential form of family connection. These family connections were integral in sustaining the family unit, providing the opportunity for children to observe family values, which are an important step in establishing identity and eventual independence. Another important aspect of the dining room table was discussion regarding family plans for the future. Holidays, visits to friends and relatives, decisions regarding family member chores, and general reminiscing about family member's daily experiences all happened at the dining room table. The family dining table was the epicenter for doing arts and crafts, making cookies, doing homework and school projects, and playing a huge variety of family games. The dining room table was a place where children could learn table manners and how to act with politeness. These essential family discussions are extremely helpful as toddlers, children and young teens explore the often confusing path of forming their own identities.

You Are What You Do

The rise in popularity of violent and sexualized television and video games, as well as reality-based television shows, reflects a surprisingly bizarre and worrisome shift in societal and cultural values. Children are very "visual", and will remember and store absolutely everything they watch in vivid visual images, converted later into long term memory. When children spend endless time watching television or playing video games, this is who they become as they begin to form their fragile and vulnerable self identities. Children with a strong sense of who they are, and what they want in life, also have a well developed personality and are less likely to need to "escape" to the world of virtual reality. In fact, children who are engaged in a variety of stimulating activities, as opposed to the narrow world of television, video games and internet, often don't understand or "get the point" of video games or reality based television programs.

A child who is only exposed to the virtual reality of television and video games, on the other hand, generally has a fragile self concept with poor self esteem, as they see the fictional characters on the screen as somehow more capable than themselves. These children adopt the identity of the character they are watching or playing, for the duration of the show or game, but when the device gets turned off, they don't really know who they are. These characters become the child's "hero", especially when the child has a poor relationship with their parents, and is unable or unwilling to model their parent's behavior. This explains to some degree our 21st century fixation with celebrities. We surround ourselves (virtually) with seemingly beautiful and flawless people, to whom we think we don't hold a candle to in comparison. So we escape into the celebrity world and wish we were them, well maybe just for a day. This type of wishful thinking is not good for our children, because the transition from the virtual world back to reality is too harsh for children to adapt to and cope.

My son had a growing addiction to television and video games when he was about 12 years old, and consequently I cancelled the cable and grossly restricted his "box" time. While my son (and all of his friends) despised me at the time, he is now a well adjusted 29 year old with a wonderful career and loads of friends, and he doesn't hold it against me. My daughter who is 16 years old has never experienced television, although she does watch the occasional movie. She plays guitar, and spends up to 20 hours a week at a local ranch with her horse, participating in equestrian competitions in the summer. While I'm far from the perfect parent, by limiting technology and directing my two children to outdoor activities, they have managed to establish solid self identities and well developed personalities, and they don't hate me for it either! Parents might think their children *want* to watch endless television and video games, but really what those children would prefer is their parent's endless and undivided attention. I've been told this fact by children many times over.

Concerns of a Grandmother

From a personal experience I have seen some of the impact that technology has had on my Step Grandchild. I have also observed children in the community on buses who appear to be oblivious of their surroundings because they have heads and eyes down in a technological device and it appeared to me that these children were being denied the opportunity to engage in the world around them.

My Grandson is now 11 years old. I first met this child when he was 5 year old. From the very first day I met him he had a technological game in his hand. He was not interested in socializing with my husband and I, my first impressions was he did not appear to have socializing skills. I found that he was oblivious to the sensory world around him; all he wanted to do was play his video game or watch TV. This behavior was troublesome for me. This unsociable behavior was even more evident when he started school. His teacher discussed her concerns with his parents and they became alarmed and concerned about the anti-social behavior. The parents decided to monitor the amount of time he was spending on the computer games, game boy etc because he was even playing game boy at recess in the school yard. The parents found that the amount of time he was involved in the use of technology was surprising and it was more than the recommended amount. His parents then decided to limit and control the amount of time he was able to have access to and on technological devices.

When they first started to limit the access to technology he became aggressive, petulant and very whinny. He kept saying he was bored, he did not know what to do. However with patience and persistence from the parents who engaged him family activities and involved him sport activities outside the home, changes in behavior began to occur. To date - he is more sociable, he has developed friendships with his peers, and he will interact with adults. But, even now when he is watching TV, on the computer, or playing game boy, he is oblivious to others in his presence and blocks out everyone and everything in the immediate environment.

Because of these observations if anyone asks me does technology affect the developing child, I say yes, I believe that technology can affect the development of socializing skills of children. I also believe that technology has its place in society but it should not take the place of parent and child interactions or, be used as a surrogate child minder. Finally, too much isolation from family members and peers is not good because too much use of technological devices can lead to anti-social behavior. Technology use denies children the opportunity to understand the world around them.

Anonymously Submitted

Chapter 9

Decline of the School Empire

Words of Wisdom from an Educational Psychologist

Since I first started writing critically about children's electronic media (around 1990) I have been continually frustrated by the laissez-faire attitudes of parents and professionals as well as the lack of substantive research on new technologies' effects on brain development. Some of this is due to ignorance and hugely expensive promotion campaigns by the media industry; much resistance has been a result of the fact that keeping kids from this truly addictive stuff is simply hard work for stressed-out parents. It is a lot easier to believe that something new and jazzy is making one's child smarter, when in fact it may well be eroding skills of thinking, attention, motivation, and language development.

Now I believe people are finally getting worried. In my book, Different Learners, I explain how excess media use, along with other aspects of children's lifestyles today, is contributing to a staggering rise in learning disabilities, social and emotional problems. Fortunately, I am also able to recommend specific steps for managing media so that it enhances rather than damages kids' mental abilities. These technologies can have positive as well as negative effects. We should be spending a lot more effort understanding and utilizing their positive potential.

Jane M. Healy, Ph.D. Educational Psychologist, Well Known Speaker and Author, Colorado

Early Intervention and Kindergrind

An interesting joint study was recently released by the British Columbia Business Council, and University of British Columbia researchers with *Human Early Learning Partnership* program, showing that just under 30% of children entering kindergarten are "developmentally vulnerable" – lacking in those basic skills they need to thrive in school and in the future. This study, entitled *A Comprehensive Policy Framework for Early Human Capital Investment in BC* states "Economic analyses reveal this depletion (in human capital) will cause British Columbia to forgo 20% of their Gross Domestic Product growth over the next 60 years, costing the provincial economy a sum of money that is ten times the total provincial debt load."

One of the authors, Dr. Paul Kershaw, said those children identified as being developmentally vulnerable as they enter kindergarten are less likely to go on and pass their foundation skills assessment test in grades 4 and 7, and more likely to not show up to even write their tests. "We know from statistical linking," Kershaw said, "that people who do badly in these tests more often than not don't go on to university. The more children that are less school-ready, the more they are less job-ready." Kershaw went on to state "The most effective use of educational funds to stimulate the economy would be to invest in the early years, even before kindergarten, when children's work and study habits are most malleable." Among its recommendations the report calls for extended parental leave, a redefinition of full-time work to accommodate shorter annual working hour norms, and increased affordable daycare.

In short, this study concludes that if parents were home more, children would get whatever it is they need to not be "developmentally vulnerable," and would pass their tests and go on to become productive members of society. With all due respect, what Dr. Kershaw and his colleges fail to consider is that while stay at home parents might be in the home, this does not mean they are available to interact with nor teach their children necessary school entry skills. Many parents are "plugged in" and "tuned out", as evidenced by studies showing internet addiction is now the fastest growing adult mental health disorder (Block, 2008). Parents are also plagued with rising levels of obesity just as are their children, and sedentary parents simply cannot provide the motor and sensory stimulation their children need for pre-literacy skill training, at least not while they are watching television or hooked into *Second Life* avatar games.

Another consideration regarding possible contributing factors to child "developmental vulnerability" is full day kindergarten, a recent mandate by British Columbia's education government. What our well meaning government fails to understand is the basics of child development. The job of the infant, toddler and preschooler is to move, a lot, experts state 2-3 hours per day of unrestricted rough and tumble play (NASPE, 2008). This constant movement provides essential sensory and motor stimulation needed to meet critical milestones for development, a precursor for attention ability and literacy. Putting children in desks and expecting them to hold a crayon is developmentally too advanced for many pre-school children, as Dr. Kershaw's 2009 study confirmed, and will only result in that child feeling performance anxiety and failure as they struggle to keep up in a world that is too difficult for them.

Anytime a child spends at a desk or with a computer in the formative early years is adversely affecting their sensory and motor development. North American education governments would be wise to look at education policies in countries such as Iceland and Finland, which have the highest literacy rates in the world. In *Smart Moves*, a book by Carla Hannaford, she states that Iceland and Finland have outdoor schools (roof, no walls) where children play on a variety of suspended equipment designed to enhance sensory and motor development. Only when children are *developmentally ready*, at the end of grade one, do these schools have children sit in desks and teach printing and reading. Progressive schools across North America are jumping on the "move to learn" bandwagon and switching to standing desks, daily treadmill use, and enforced outdoor recess.

Exposing children to more structured education, does not necessarily equate to improved literacy and learning skill as the United States found out with their "No Child Left Behind" education initiatives launched during the George Bush era. We learned from Dr. Kershaw's study that children who enter school developmentally delayed do not "catch up". Governments might consider focusing early intervention efforts at the daycare and pre-school level, where environments could be re-structured to include some of the Iceland and Finland sensory and motor enhancing components, discussed in greater detail in Section II. We are raising children, not little adults. Every child has the right to literacy, but "too much too soon" removes that right.

"Educational" Computers?

With the rise in computer use in the school setting, I was interested to hear student perceptions regarding computer use in actual school settings. I interviewed elementary and high school students and teachers in my school district regarding use of technology in their schools, and discovered some interesting information. Students are frequently allowed unrestricted and unsupervised access to their school's computer lab during school hours, recess, lunch time, and before/after school, although not in all schools, and not all students. While one might assume students are doing school work during this time, apparently they are not (refer to below comments). Playing computer games appears to occupy the majority of in-school computer use time, although this much repeated fact was apparently not known by school staff or parents. Another interesting note was that in one school, all grade 3-7 students had been provided with their own laptops, yet the grade 8-12's were expected to share a bank of 15 laptops amongst the lot of them. One student actually stated to me "What would a grade 3 do with a computer!" Texting on cell phones and listening to iPods during class, are other challenges facing today's education professionals.

The following comments are from interviews with elementary students from a school on the Sunshine Coast in British Columbia:

- "We do a bunch of projects on computers, and it takes us away from other work. Like – we haven't done math in 2 weeks, and no French in 3 weeks."
- "Some of my friends were getting straight A's and now their not. Sometimes they say they can't concentrate, but I'm not really sure what that's about."
- "We get a lot of work to do on computers, and we don't go outside as much as we used to. I choose to do school work on the computers, but most kids just play games. When students work in pairs on projects, stuff doesn't get done because they are playing games."
- "Everyone thinks computers make kids smarter, but I think computers make kids dumber. They (computers) keep changing and changing and changing."
- "Any time they want, kids can get on the computer, but they just play games. Three of them got their computer confiscated because of a "chat" thing, but they just watch others now. They use one hand to eat, and the other to play."

These student comments bring to light an interesting problem in the education sector – how do education professionals keep up with the times, but also ensure children achieve literacy and academic success? Schools are receiving pressure from parents to provide their children with new age technology, yet are also reporting that their children can't print and read. Could it be that technology use and attainment of literacy are mutually exclusive? What resources are available to guide schools through this transition time of attempting to accommodate the technology explosion?

My experience has been that no one is even *questioning* the "ramping up" of technology usage in the school setting. To my knowledge there are no regulatory guidelines for limiting or managing technology use in school settings. Possible areas of consideration regarding use of personal technology in school would be:

- Use of computers for non-school related activities e.g. gaming;
- Use of cell phones and iPods in classrooms;
- Closure of computer lab when lack of staffing prohibits adequate supervision e.g. during lunch, recess and before/after school;
- Support and promotion of student participation in organized sports on the playground.

Computers vs. Playgrounds – It's a No Brainer!

Teachers report with increasing frequency that playgrounds are in a state of disrepair, while school expenditures on technology routinely exceed budget allocations. Year after year research shows that exercise makes kids smarter and technology doesn't (Ratey, 2008, Healy, 2010), yet schools continue to invest in technology at the detriment of child health and literacy. Why is this? The rapidity with which technology has entered the home and school system is staggering, and allows little time for parents or teachers to critically analyze what is really happening to their children. What has been known for decades is that children need to move to learn, and when movement is restricted by allowing technology to replace recess and lunch in outdoor playground areas, children can't learn. It is really that simple. Schools need to manage a balance between achieving critical elements for child growth and success, with use of technology.

Access to playgrounds during recess and lunch offers children a variety of types of movement, as well as ample opportunity to socialize and participate in creative and imaginary play. Yet, many schools allow children to stay inside and "work" on computers during recess and lunch, often unsupervised, detrimentally affecting their health, development and academic performance. Unstructured play in a nature based environment provides *attention restoration* necessary for optimal brain productivity (Kuo, 2000). Sitting for extended periods gazing at a two-dimensional screen fine tuning the art of killing, actually "short circuits" the frontal cortex, eliminating executive function altogether, as well as destroys impulse control making it virtually impossible to attend or learn (Small, 2007). Schools allowing playground equipment to become antiquated and in disrepair is not only unconscionable, but also short sighted, resulting in failed literacy and unmanageable behaviors.

What do children need for optimal development and productivity, and how can playground equipment meet those needs? Children need adequate sensory input to their vestibular, proprioceptive, and tactile sensory systems in order to achieve optimal core posture, bilateral coordination of the body and eyes, and praxis – or ability to perform planned movement patterns. Posture, coordination and praxis form the foundation for all fine and gross motor activities, such as printing, reading and sports. Engagement in 2-3 hours per day of unstructured rough and tumble play ensures children get the type of activity they need to grow and succeed. Playground structures are an integral component for attaining literacy, as they ensure children meet critical developmental milestones necessary for eventual printing and reading. Yet – their very children who need this sensory and motor development, are the ones kept inside at recess to finish their work! Playground structures should contain elements that contribute to the development of the vestibular, proprioceptive and tactile sensory systems. Sensory and motor system development is covered extensively in Section II, as is "sensational" playground design.

Children are our future, and there is no future in the unconscious use of technology. Curtailing or freezing technology expenditures, and diverting this money toward upgrading gyms, classrooms and playground equipment, will result in immediate improvements in children's ability to attend and learn. Technology awareness programs that teach children how to manage balanced technology use, will result in reductions in child aggression and obesity, as well as long term improvements in literacy and academic performance.

Not Teach Printing???

I was consulting in northern British Columbia in a remote First Nations community, and was working with a bright and energetic grade four student who had been referred for "learning difficulties". The resource teacher stated that she thought this student was underperforming, and had this year exhibited significant defiance and difficult behavior. I was observing this child doing his math sheet, and when he looked at me and asked if the number he just printed was a "5" (it looked a bit more like a backward "7" to me), I realized he didn't know how to print. I asked the resource teacher to scribe for this child, and he literally jumped to the challenge and proceeded to fly through progressively harder math sheets getting all correct answers. Here was a delightful, smart and extremely frustrated child trapped in a system that had not taught him how to print.

I would like to ask readers to perform a short exercise to help illustrate how children who are not taught to print feel on a minute by minute basis in our schools. Write or print your name. Now do the same, only do it mirror image backward. Now write or print this way for the next week. How do you feel right now, having been given a task with minimal instruction which you neither knew how to complete nor had the skill to do so? Confused, frustrated a bit defiant? If you were required to do this exercise indefinitely, you might even eventually develop "behavior problems". For adults, this approach to non-teaching would be similar to signing up for a class in learning how to write in Hebrew, or Chinese, but showing up and there is no teacher – but there will be an exam! Hopefully, somehow on your own, you would eventually develop a "motor plan" for this new way of producing written output, but that's because you are an intelligent adult with average motor skills, and not a developmentally delayed child, as 30% of our primary children are today (Kershaw, 2009).

Declining interest by educators to teaching printing skills continues to astound me. When children's grades in the elementary setting are based largely on output produced by printing, one would think that some effort to teach this essential skill would be warranted. Instead, far too often, lack of printing skill is perceived as a "learning disability" when really it is a "teaching disability", and the consolation prize is to hand children who can't print a computer.

Literacy On a Dime

I recently completed a six week pilot project designed to enhance literacy and printing skills in two school kindergarten classrooms on the Sunshine Coast in British Columbia. This project consisted of the following components:

1. Develop a screening tool for kindergartners to identify sensory and motor components that limit acquiring literacy.
2. Design a 3 hour teacher workshop on methods to promote literacy.
3. Design and pilot test twelve twice weekly pull-out sessions to enhance attention, gross motor, oculomotor, fine motor, visual motor, praxis, and hand function skill components.
4. Perform a final evaluation using initial screening tool.

Approximately 30% of each classroom was identified as developmentally delayed and subsequently referred for intervention by resource and classroom teachers, a statistic congruent with Paul Kershaw's 2009 study findings. Results of the initial screening indicated that the students all demonstrated exceptionally poor spatial concepts and inability to pay attention. Classroom observation indicated that the teachers lacked consistency of rules for printing, and had no wall surface for teaching printing (chalk or white boards) instead of using table tops. Following the implementation of this pull-out program in two schools, results of my pilot study indicated 12% and 18% overall improvements in pre-literacy skills in the two schools, with 29% and 26% improvements in hand function, and 16% and 26% improvements in visual motor skills (the two most significant skill deficit areas).

While this pilot project was just a start toward a far more expansive pre-literacy program, it illustrated that a minimal intervention (two ½ hour weekly sessions) can go a long way toward improving children's ability to print. At this crucial point in time, when educators are actively making the decision to not teach printing skills, and instead turning the job of literacy over to computers, they would be wise to ask the question "Where is the evidence that supports this choice?" I have long and hard championed the return of printing as a curriculum-based subject with all our Canadian provincial Education Ministries. If printing were curriculum-based, researchers could determine the best methods of teaching and evaluation, and teacher colleges and universities would include this much needed information for their new teachers. If printing were curriculum-based, teachers would provide consistent and adequate instruction for students to easily achieve literacy in the primary grades.

The Myth of Computer Efficiency

A high school teacher recently told me that following installation of a "new and improved" computerized operating system in her school, it took her 2.5 hours to change one student's grade. This teacher longed for the days of "pencil and eraser," and stated computers are "The bane of my existence; I don't even use email!" While this teacher might be a rarity, her experience of frustration regarding the "ever changing" computer system is not. How many of us have experienced absolute "meltdowns" regarding learning a new computer program, or trying to repair a non-functioning one? Teacher time spent on computers is time taken away from students. No matter how justifiable a new program might be, based largely on promises from the manufacturer, students still need their teachers.

Frustrations of a School Counselor

This past year has not been a very satisfactory one in our local high school. The implementation of a new on-line "records collecting" program has limited the amount of time that counselors have for face to face direct contact with students. The software has not made our jobs easier but rather more cumbersome and time consuming so that we have even less time to speak to students directly about any issues that they may be experiencing.

Emotional issues (at the high school level) get put on the back burner, as counselors attempt to get kids scheduled so that the daily routine of classes can unfold. Because of the inefficiencies of the software program, it takes much longer to get all the students scheduled into their first choice classes. So we spend a lot of time with students in our offices looking at a computer screen together (rather than at each other) in an attempt to get students into their classes.

Because of the issues with this new program, time spent on the computer trying to balance classes and schedules has increased by at least 3 times. In other words, if we counselors used to spend 3 hrs per day on average on the computer dealing with the technological side of timetabling, this time has increased by 3 times. Therefore, our computer time per day has gone up to about 9 hours, in theory.

Obviously, we do not spend, 9 hours per day at the office, let alone in front of our computers. But this "clunky" software translates into a certain change in the atmosphere in the counseling office. When students arrive at our office door, they can immediately sense the level of tension and urgency that is in the air. When they ask if we are busy, they already know the answer: "That we are ALWAYS busy".

However, if and when students arrive with an emotional issue, my colleague and I always put aside the technological stuff in order to focus on the emotional. We almost jump at the chance to help students who dare to come forward with emotional things. This is happening less and less frequently, as students pick up on the atmosphere in our office. They do not want to disturb us, as we attempt to get all the technological glitches that need resolving at any semester change.

In other words, the use of technology in our offices has changed how we respond to students' emotional needs. I believe that the school's focus on technology has reduced the number of students who come to the counseling office for guidance Re; their emotional concerns.

Deborah Alain, Art Therapist and High School Counselor, British Columbia.

SECTION II

Requirement - Critical Factors for Child Development

Looking at Both Sides of the Coin – Mother of a Child with Sensory Processing Disorder

We have a child with severe dyspraxia. He has spent over five thousand hours since the age of 4 working on the "Handwriting Without Tears Program" in hopes of getting him to write. He is about to turn 10 and to date can't write without a template. However give him a computer, and he is typing words and creating sentences. Technology has been his way of entering into the educational world allowing him equal playing field.

Having said that, what we have seen is technology seems to be going the "other way". We are losing human connection in the school systems and at home. A multi-sensory approach, human touch, human voice, connection eye to eye, is leaving our school systems and being replaced with digital teaching.

At home we have noticed that when we allow our children to "download" and watch t.v. and or play on the computer, the opposite is what occurs, they don't download and become regulated, they get supercharged and "amped" up. With having Sensory Processing Disorder, how my children react to technology is like watching a diabetic get too much sugar. When we cut back their t.v. time and computer time and replace it with games we play at the table and games outside, we see calmer children who are paying greater attention and whose SPD becomes more manageable.

Although technology is a gift, it like everything else needs to be in balance, and should never be a way to replace human contact and connection from the teacher in our school systems. It makes me very concerned that our children are going to be labeled more and more and receive more medications to get them to sit and attend while we put more and more stimulators in front of them. Yet at the same time we are reducing times in the classroom for movement and time to allow the children to regulate their nervous systems.

Lori Fankhanel, mother of two exceptional children and
President of *Sensory Processing Disorder Canada Foundation*, Alberta.

Foundations for Development

In times past, through play and social interaction, children received necessary sensory and motor stimulation to develop properly. When they got to school, they had established pre-literacy skills foundation essential for paying attention and learning. This is no longer the case in 21st century children.

A Psychologist's Views on Electronic Media

When a child is using the electronic media, they are not engaged in physical interaction with the environment or social interaction. Throughout childhood, but in the early years in particular, physical activity is an essential ingredient for healthy development. Not only of the body, but also of the brain and nerve pathways involved in control of balance, eye movements needed to support reading and writing, and body and spatial awareness.

Physical activity and social engagement help to develop the ability to read body language (non-verbal language) of others and to regulate and adapt response. Up to 90% of effective communication is based on the non-verbal nuances of language such as posture, gesture, eye contact, tone of voice and rate of speech, Children who spend many hours playing with computer games are not developing these crucial social skills.

Computer programs tend to be developed by people with a particular type of brain functioning. Many hours exposed to these programs may help to "shape" the developing brain in one particular direction to the detriment of other skills.

Sally Goddard Blythe, Director of the *Institute for Neuro-Physiological Psychology* and Author, UK.

Chapter 10

A Cracked Foundation

I've completed a number of courses in the area of child development, attachment theory, as well as have my certification in *Sensory Integration and Praxis*. What I have learned thus far is that raising a child is like building a house, it's all about the foundation. When building a house, the foundation needs to be constructed properly for optimal longevity and integrity. The materials need to be made of high quality ingredients, and the contactor and construction crews need to be knowledgeable and experienced. There are critical time factors that need to be adhered to, and proper preparation and planning ensures smooth and uneventful construction. Crews need to get along and be properly compensated to keep everyone happy and productive. When any of the aforementioned factors are faulty or inadequate, so will be the foundation, threatening the overall structure and sustainability of the house.

When raising a child, prior preparation and planning by prospective parents will ensure adequate knowledge and experience for child health and safety. Child growth and development have numerous critical periods which need to be met on a timely basis. While food, shelter, and clothing are all essential ingredients for raising a healthy child, so are other critical elements of adequate movement, touch and human connection. As family life is stressful, members need to work together and support the family unit. When any of the aforementioned factors are faulty or inadequate, so will be the foundation, threatening the overall structure and sustainability of the child.

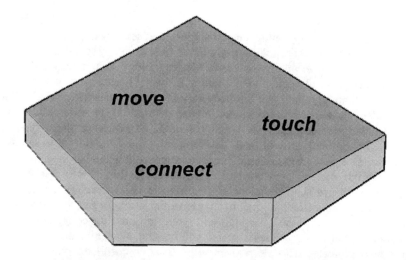

The underlying premise of both *Virtual Child* and occupational therapy is that children need adequate amounts of critical factors for development, namely movement, touch and connection with other humans. These critical factors then enable the child to attain optimal physical, mental, social and academic performance. Failure to receive these critical components results in child mal-development, and a host of disorders that the health and education systems are just beginning to detect. Our experts are barely starting to study these deficits, never mind provide extensive evidence-based interventions. Frequent movement by infants, toddlers and children establishes essential postural tone and coordination of the muscles of the body and eyes. These developmental milestones are integral for eventual school readiness for printing and reading. Movement also helps a child maintain optimal arousal states for paying attention and learning. Adequate touch helps a child to know where their body is in space, and is important for helping a child to feel calm and relaxed. A child who is deprived of touch exhibits anxiety, fear and has difficulty adapting to any new environment or situation. Human connection is a *biological need* without which children die. Social isolation from overuse of technology is resulting in children who are depressed, anxious and scared, which give rise to mental states that prohibit learning.

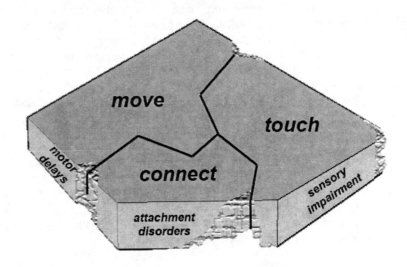

Extensive overuse of technology has finally "cracked" the foundations for child development. Motor delays, attachment disorders, and sensory impairment are the aftermath. Time spent overusing technology grossly limits time children spend in activities other than technology, resulting in an *over reliance* on technology that may eventually become an addiction. A premise of occupational therapy is that "You are what you do." If all a child does is use technology, their life becomes very limited and narrow. Pursuit of activities that promote adequate movement, touch and human connection, provide children with an array of choices that broaden their skill and potential. Exposure to these types of activities necessary for optimal growth and development, allows children to attain a level of performance skill that promotes enjoyment and success in whatever they choose to do.

Current societal pressure and expectations for high performance of children are incongruent with profound deficiencies occurring in child development today. Repeatedly asking a child to do a task that they neither have the skills for nor the interest in, is a recipe for disaster. Setting the "bar" too high will erode self confidence and esteem, two integral components for mental wellness, social ability, and academic performance. Supporting research now indicates technology overuse by children correlates with increased incidence of the following conditions: aggression, anxiety, depression, adhd, poor academic performance, obesity, delayed development, motor coordination disorder, sensory processing disorder, and early sexuality. The foundation for child development has finally cracked, and the damage may, at this time, be beyond repair.

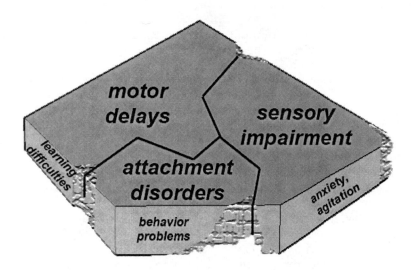

The Human Body Was Not Biologically Designed To Be Sedentary

A well accepted concept in developmental research is that children's bodies need to move to achieve optimal sensory and motor development (Ayres, 1972; Braswell, 2006). Developing children require 2 to 3 hours per day of unstructured, active rough-and-tumble play to achieve adequate stimulation to the vestibular, proprioceptive, and tactile sensory systems to optimize development and learning (National Association for Sport and Physical Education, 2002; Ayres, 1972; Pelligrini, 2005; Tannock, 2008). This type of sensory and motor input ensures normal development of a child's core posture, bilateral coordination, and optimal arousal states necessary for eventual development of pre-literacy skills (Rine, 2004). Infants with low tone, toddlers failing to reach motor milestones, and children who are unable to pay attention or achieve basic sensory and motor foundation skills for literacy are now the norm. These are the children who are now frequent visitors to pediatric physiotherapy, occupational therapy, and speech and language therapy clinics.

Playgrounds, once the epicenter for child play and interaction, have either fallen into disrepair, or are so infantile in skill requirements that only the smallest of the toddler set are challenged. I am routinely informed by my workshop participants, that many schools are deciding to upgrade their computers, at the expense of allowing their playgrounds to fall apart. Children need to move in order to develop sensory and motor components necessary to learn. Removing the playground equipment prohibits this essential skill development. One special education teacher informed me that her principal had actually cordoned off the school playground with yellow tape, yet this same school's computer lab had received three upgrades to *all* of their 30 computers in one year's budget. This is a school who will not only be dealing with developmental delays and literacy issues, but their student's behavior issues are likely to be off the map in a very short time.

While it is widely known that increased activity reduces obesity and enhances child development, many children who are obese or developmentally delayed do not have the motor skills, agility, nor the confidence needed to play on traditional playgrounds. So – many of these disadvantaged children either spend their breaks in the computer lab, or just stand around during recess using a growing variety of hand held technological devices. Parents who perceive outdoor play as "unsafe" allow children higher usages of technology, further limiting access to developmental components usually attained in outdoor rough-and-tumble playground play (Burdette & Whitaker, 2006).

Imbalanced Sensation

Children require a variety of balanced sensations in order to grow and develop into healthy and happy individuals. The advent of technology has resulted in a *sensory deprived* world for many children, a world where children don't need to move anymore to survive. Biologically, the human body was designed to perform physical "heavy work" type activities, not be sedentary. As human systems have devolved to cater to the lazy, unmotivated adult, we errantly began to think that it was okay that children don't move either. This ill founded belief is the major reason why we are drugging so many children…we are expecting them to become sedentary right along with us adults. We have forgotten that children need to *move*, as well as be exposed to a variety of other sensations, to grow up healthy and be able to learn.

Lack of movement is having a significant negative impact on normal sensory and motor system development, and is creating huge problems not only with delays in development, but also with child behavior management at home and in schools as well. But getting children to *move more* is not the only answer. Optimal child development happens when a child is exposed to a *balance* of sensory input from the environment through their senses e.g. touch, movement, smell, taste, auditory, visual. Balanced sensory input then allows the child to integrate and make sense of this information. Termed "sensory integration", balanced sensory input helps a child to choose an appropriate or functional output, which could be a motor or muscle act, or how the child feels or behaves. Functional sensory processing and integration enable a child to ultimately pay attention and learn.

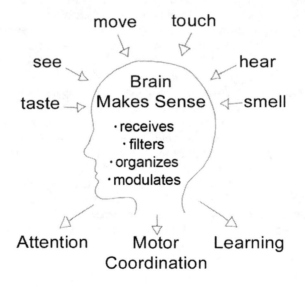

Children who spend a lot of time with technology receive too much auditory and visual stimulation, and too little touch and movement stimulation. This creates an imbalanced sensory system, and results in delays in motor development, attention and learning. This concept of sensory integration will be covered in more detail in subsequent chapters, and will form the groundwork for recommendations made for changes to our home, school and community environments.

Chapter 11

Child Developmental Milestones

Whether a parent or a teacher, it is important to know the developmental level of a child in order to know if there is indeed a developmental delay and need for further intervention. Often determining developmental level requires the assistance of a trained professional such as a pediatric occupational therapist, physical therapist or speech and language pathologist. Unfortunately, pediatric therapists are stretched pretty thin in the school setting these days. In light of recent research showing 30% of children entering kindergarten developmentally delayed, the pre-school, daycare and primary teachers are required to gain knowledge in the area of assessing developmental level, in order to ensure each child receives *developmentally*, not *age appropriate* instruction. Once a child's level of development is determined, then steps can be taken in the right direction to improve development through provision of appropriate programming. This developmental approach in the education system is essential if we are ever to begin to address the profound developmental "gap" we are seeing in schools today.

I would like to offer a brief overview of normal child development, which is a necessary contrast point in helping parents and education professionals understand the extent of child developmental delays. I have designed the following two *Foundation Scales* for use in daycare, pre-school and school based settings:

- *The Foundation Scale for Infants, Toddlers and Pre-School Children*
- *The Foundation Scale for Grades K - Seven Children*

These two scales were formulated through collation of information from a number of infant, toddler and child sensory, motor and speech resource tools, as well as reviews of relevant research literature, Canadian curriculum guidelines, and consultation from pediatric therapists and resource teachers. These scales are "approximate" only, and therefore should not be interpreted as accurate or predictive. These *Foundation Scales* should not be used for research purposes.

The purpose for these two scales are as *guides* to assist parents and teachers in determining if their children are meeting age and grade level expectations. These skills should be achieved by the *end* of the relevant age.

Foundation Scale for Infant, Toddler and Preschool Children

Age	Posture and Coordination	Crawling and Stairs	Eyes and Hands	Self Care	Speech	Socialization
3 mos.	Controls head Tries to roll		Eyes track parent	Swallows soft foods	Smiles Sounds communicate pleasure and discomfort	Sustains eye contact Calms when parent present
6 mos.	Sits without support for 5 mins.	Bum scoot	Palm down grasp	Controls lips	Waves	Interacts with parent Imitates parent facial gestures
9 mos.	Stands without support	Crawls without rhythm	Full arc eye movements	Drinks with assistance	Says one word Understands "no"	Returns affection Intentional gestures
12 mos.	Walks with support	Rhythmic crawling Tries to crawl up stairs	Thumb up grasp Scribbles	Positions limbs when dressing Pees in potty	Says three words Communicate with gestures	Responds to simple requests Expresses (& represses) desires
18 mos.	Walks without support Stands on one foot	Climbs stairs with stand by support	Holds and looks at book Draws random lines	Drinks with sippy cup Swallows solid foods	Two word sentences	Stranger anxiety and separation anxiety evident
2 years	Jumps with both feet Walks backward	Climbs stairs facing rail	Turns pages of book Tip to tip grasp Draws vertical line	Attempts utensil use Assists with dressing Poos in potty	Sings simple repetitive song lyrics	Attempts social rules "thank you", "please" Dress up play Dances to music
3 years	Catches object with arms and body Controlled running Rides tricycle	Climbs stairs facing forward using rail, one foot at a time	Cuts object with scissors Scissors often upside down Draws circle	Dresses self except socks, tying shoes and fasteners Toilet trained for daytime; assistance for wiping	Three word sentences Indicates own age with fingers	Reciprocal conversations Curious; asks questions Asserts self

4 years	Catches object with both hands Skips uncontrolled Rides bike with training wheels	Climbs stairs using rail, alternating feet	Pretend reading Stabilizes paper with one hand while cutting with other Correct scissor position Draws horizontal lines	Accomplish utensil use Dresses self except for tying shoes and some fasteners Toilet trained for day and night time; attempts wiping	Four words sentences	Knows and is able to anticipate consequences of own actions Waits turn for tasks 4 min. attention on task of choice
5 years	Catches object with one hand Controlled skipping Rides bike	Climbs stairs without rail, alternating feet Controlled skipping	Reads 2-3 words Cuts circle shape Draws diagonal lines Makes shapes	Attempts knife cutting Dresses self except for some fasteners Independent toileting and wiping	Five word sentences	Waits turn in conversation without interrupting 5 min. attention on task of choice

Foundation Scale for Grades K - Seven Children

Grade	Age	Printing	Spelling	Reading	Attention
Pre-K	4-5 years	Strokes, shapes, simple drawings; writes own name	Spells own name	Recognizes own name	5 minutes sustained attention on required task
K	5-6	Some letters, some directional sense (left/right, up/down) Prints 8.5 letters per minute in a copy task	Spells words of 1-3 letters	Recognizes some 3 letter words	6 minutes attention Inhibition of impulse control matures
1	6-7	Upper and lower case letters, numbers Prints 18.9 letters per minute	Spells words up to 5 letters	Oral reads ~ 12 words per minute	7 minutes
2	7-8	Letters on the line, accurate spacing, no reversals Prints 33.9 letters per minute	Spells words up to 6-7 letters	Oral reads ~ 25 words per minute	8 minutes
3	8-9	Legible printing; starts cursive Prints 47.3 letters per minute	Spells words up to 7-8 letters	Silent reads ~ 50 words per minute	15 minutes
4	9-10	Legible cursive Cursive 63.2 letters per minute	Spells words up to 8-9 letters	Silent reads ~ 75 words per minute	20 minutes; focused attention matures
5	10-11	Cursive 72.7 letters per minute	Spells words up to 9-10 letters	Silent reads ~ 100 words per minute	25 minutes
6	11-12	Cursive 84.7 letters per minute	Spells multi-syllabic words	Silent reads ~ 150 words per minute	30 minutes
7	12-13	Cursive 99.9 letters per minute	Spells more advanced multi-syllabic words	Silent reads ~ 300 words per minute (~ 1/3 page)	45 minutes

Developmental Hierarchy

In building foundations for optimal child development, it's wise to think in terms of a developmental hierarchy based on the needs and requirements of the child at different stages in development. In my role and area of expertise as a pediatric occupational therapist, I will restrict my discussion to the requirements of the developing child for aspects related to the development of the sensory, motor and attachment systems. Other systems should be taken into consideration when determining a comprehensive, overall developmental picture for a child. I will begin this section by discussing aspects pertaining to sensory, motor and attachment development.

Chapter 12

Sensory and Motor Development

A bit of basic neurology is necessary to help readers better understand concepts regarding sensory and motor system development. This information will also serve to allow readers the necessary background information to apply effective sensory and motor tools and techniques to enhance development and learning ability. To achieve normal sensory and motor system development, children need stimulation and integration of the vestibular, tactile and proprioceptive sensory channels which work together to mediate movement and touch (refer to *Sensory and Motor Development* diagram below). Integration of sensory channels in the first stage of development is a precursor to being able to learn through the more advanced auditory and visual sensory channels which mediate hearing and vision in Stage 2. Only when Stage 1 movement and touch sensory channels become integrated, can a child process through their Stage 2 hearing and vision channels, essential for academic learning in Stage 3.

This sensory input is critical from early infancy, toddler and childhood, and needs to be balanced and of adequate duration for optimal development to occur. Children who overuse technology have too much sensory input to the auditory and visual channels, and too little sensory input into the vestibular, tactile and proprioceptive (movement and touch) channels. This sensory imbalance results in suboptimal development and consequent impairments in attention and learning ability.

Sensory and Motor System Development

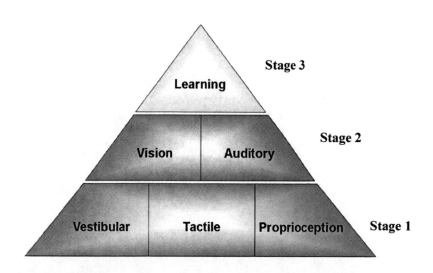

The *vestibular system* is the foundation for all other sensory systems, and is integral in the development of posture, coordination and arousal states. Poor vestibular function results in a child who either moves constantly or fears movement, and has either sleepy or hyper energy. The *proprioceptive system* promotes optimal muscle tone and strength, allowing a child to *grade* fine and gross motor movement. Children who have difficulty grading movements are always bumping into things, and seem clumsy. The *tactile system* determines a child's ability to plan *purposeful* movements. A child with tactile sensory dysfunction often will touch everything or have an aversive response to touch, and may appear anxious or agitated.

Think of babies and how they learn. They move constantly by crawling about to explore their world, putting everything in their mouth. These actions stimulate the vestibular, tactile and proprioceptive sensory channels, promoting optimal development. Young children continue to require Stage 1 sensory stimulation throughout the elementary years in order to adequately process information through their Stage 2 vision and hearing channels. This sensory stimulation allows them to ultimately attend and focus on tasks, and feel healthy and happy in everyday life.

As adults, think about what you might do on a weekend or an evening that makes you feel good and able to be productive at work the next day. Digging in the garden, playing sports, taking the dog for a long walk, and working out in the gym are some examples of vestibular and proprioceptive sensory input. Snuggling on the couch, play wrestling with your kids, hugging, and getting a massage are all examples of tactile sensory input that helps us to feel calm and relaxed. Alternatively, think about how productive you were at work, or how lousy you felt, when you just sat around alone in your house all evening or on the weekend, watching television or movies, or spending long periods at the computer? Technology has virtually eliminated our need to move and touch, and not only our children, but also our adult populations are showing signs of *sensory deprivation* with stress related illnesses and subsequent absenteeism. Anti-depressant and stress medication use is higher than it has ever been for adults and children, as they strive to adapt to our sedentary yet fast paced, immediate, technology loaded world.

Let's talk more specifically about the vestibular, proprioceptive and tactile sensory systems, and how these systems can work together to enable pre-literacy skills and allow child to pay attention and learn. When readers understand these three systems, they will begin to grasp how technology deprives children of essential elements for development, and works to limit learning potential.

Movement

Readers may have watched a recent movie called "Wall-E" where humans live on a space ship because their earth planet was no longer habitable due to piles of garbage. These humans lye about on motorized lounge chairs, and are waited on by flying robots who bring them drink, food etc. Because they never move, these humans are quite obese and during one funny scene, one human fell off his lounge chair and not only couldn't get up, but had forgotten how to walk! As a result of not moving, these futuristic humans relied on robotic assistance for even the most mundane of tasks. Of course, the Captain of the space ship eventually teaches himself how to walk again, and saves the day, as well as all his passengers. While this movie was produced for children, it has a poignant message for adults as well.

This section will discuss why movement is so important for child health and academic performance, and how different types of movement not only ensure health, but also promote literacy. New age technologies are forever changing the ways in which we move through our world, at great detriment to human health and well being.

Chapter 13

The Vestibular System

My son actually seems to fear movement. He hates going up or down stairs or walking over uneven ground, and forget swings, slides or playgrounds...they make him scream. His feet never seem to leave the ground, and he refuses to run or jump. He holds his head in this downward position all the time, and never looks up.

My daughter craves movement, and never stops. We call her the "energizer bunny". She seems so clumsy though, always falling down and bumping into things. She always seems to be dragging her feet on the floor, and runs everywhere. She has this burst of speed, and then gets tired so quickly. She holds her head in this rigid position, like it's going to fall off her neck. What does this mean?

These are familiar comments by parents of children who have difficulty processing and integrating information from their vestibular system. These children often "seek" vestibular stimulation through movement, or "avoid" vestibular stimulation by holding still. This allows them to organize their arousal state, necessary for paying attention and learning.

Where is the Vestibular System Located?

The vestibular system is located deep inside our brain, and is often referred to as our "inner ear", as its location is an extension of our ear apparatus. The vestibular system is made up of two apparatus, each of which has a series of semicircular canals filled with fluid that "swooshes" around each time we move our head. These canals are positioned in three different dimensional planes, thereby detecting rotational, linear and horizontal movement. The vestibular system also has unique organs called otoliths that detect *linear acceleration* and thereby work to help a child hold their head and trunk stable. Children with malfunctioning otoliths, often have difficulty stabilizing their head, often feels dizzy, and consequently raise their shoulders around their neck for increased head stability.

Children who have an underdeveloped vestibular system have poor trunk stability from weak core stabilizer muscles, resulting in generalized "low tone". Children with low tone have difficulty using both sides of the body together, called *bilateral integration*, and may experience difficulty standing on one leg, manipulating items with both hands, or playing off their body midline. Children with vestibular problems also have great difficulty coordinating eye and hand movements, as the eye muscles may not be "talking" to each other and tend to function somewhat independently. These children are also not able to regulate their arousal states, resulting in a low arousal, or hyper aroused child.

The Vestibular System

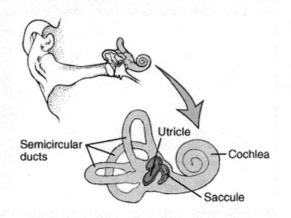

What is the Function of the Vestibular System?

The vestibular system helps children know where their body is in space, and where their body is in relationship to other people and objects. The vestibular system works through activating muscles that control postural tone, muscles that keep us upright against gravity. In order to best understand how vestibular stimulation impacts on the formation of core tone and strength, think of a child off a swing. When the swing moves forward, the gravitational forces are pushing the child backward on the swing. The child's body reacts to contract the muscles on the front side of the body in order to maintain core strength and not fall off the swing. When the swings moves in the reverse position or backward, the gravitational forces push the child forward on the swing causing contraction of the back side of the child's body. The vestibular system is always working when a child is moving, to send messages to different sets of muscles to contract to keep the child upright and maintaining core tone and posture.

The formation of core tone and upright posture is integral for the consequent formation of the coordination of the upper and lower body, right side of the body to left side, and the coordination of both eyes. Without the development of core posture, the infant, toddler, or child's trunk tone is like that of a wet noodle or "floppy", and coordination becomes impossible. Infants who lye for long periods on their backs either in cribs, or in bucket seats, are not stimulating their vestibular systems. This under stimulation is hugely detrimental to this formation of core tone and eventual motor coordination. Toddlers strapped into strollers or back packs, or being carried all the time and not allowed to walk or stumble, fall and get up, also further limit formation of core tone. Children who spend hours "schulmped" on a soft couch playing video games, or laying on their bed watching television, will have delayed vestibular development and likely have poor core stability and motor coordination.

Children who have a dysfunctional vestibular system are unable to regulate their arousal states, necessary for paying attention and learning. Think of what we do as adults to either calm or arouse an infant. If we want them to go to sleep, we either rock them, or drive them around in a car. This movement is stimulating all of the three vestibular channels, resulting in a lowering of the infant's arousal state and hopefully, eventual sleep. Alternatively, think what we do as adults to arouse a sleepy or lethargic infant. Grandma is here, and wants to see her grandchild who just woke up from a long nap. We might swing the infant back and forth or up and down to wake them up, so they'll smile and coo, and Grandma will "ooh" and "ahh". Children who don't move enough, don't receive adequate vestibular stimulation to regulate their arousal or energy states, and consequently have energy that is either too sleepy and zoned out, or too hyper and charged.

Why Children Who Don't' Move Can't Pay Attention and Learn

Functional vestibular systems require frequent movement off the center of gravity to optimize the development of core stability and motor coordination, which are integral for eventual printing and reading ability. Children who have low trunk tone and poor coordination, are unable to coordinate both sides of their body, their upper and lower body, and their eyes. Consequently these children have difficulty sitting upright in a chair to do their work. They are unable to stabilize their paper and hold a pencil to print. They can't control the muscles of their eyes to read, or coordinate their eyes with their hand to print. Most importantly, they cannot optimize their arousal states to be able to pay attention and learn. Under stimulated vestibular systems, such as are found in children who overuse technology, prevent learning.

When a child doesn't move, their vestibular system does not develop properly, or is not *integrating* with other sensory systems such as vision. The consequences are that the child may feel uncomfortable or sick, anxious and even scared, resulting in behaviors that are often difficult for parents and teachers to understand. The reason why some children refuse to close their eyes when standing, or to put their heads under water, is that they may be relying on the visual system to compensate for a malfunctioning vestibular system.

Only recently has research shed light on the integral role of movement and exercise on a child's ability to pay attention and learn. Dr. John Ratey, child psychiatrist, researcher and author of the book *Spark – The revolutionary new science of exercise and the brain*, found that not only does exercise increase circulation to the frontal cortex, which is known for executive function and impulse control, but exercise was also found to result in neurogenesis, or growth of new neurons, in the hippocampal and limbic regions in the brain, known to be essential for learning and memory. Dr. Ratey's research found that exercise consisting of 45 minutes per day using treadmills and/or exercise bikes, of sufficient intensity to raise the child's heart rate to 65-75% of its maximum, also caused a surge in dopamine, acetylcholine and serotonin transmitters, which had secondary effects of an observed reduction in child impulsivity, anxiety and depression. A systematic review of children with autism, when engaged in physical exercise, showed decreases in stereotypy, aggression, off-task behavior, and elopement (Lang, 2010).

Let's look at what has happened over the past 20 years with the explosion of media technology. For hundreds of thousands of years, human beings needed to move to survive, and movement was a large part of a child's daily existence and integral to a child's developing vestibular system. Children were often engaged in heavy work: chopping wood, hauling water, and plowing fields. During these activities, children's vestibular systems were inverted, spun around, and tipped side to side. Movement involved acceleration and rapid changes in direction, as children worked and played rough and tumble games. Now children sit for long periods inside, and if they do get out to the playground, everything seems designed for a toddler and is uninteresting, so they go back inside and play more video games.

How to Know if a Child has a Vestibular Processing Problem

Following are a list of some common traits of children with vestibular dysfunction that you can easily identify by watching children move about in their environment:

- Unable to lie on stomach and do a "Superman" e.g. arms and legs stretched out and lifted off the ground;
- Low muscle tone or weakness in trunk, neck, arms or legs;

- Unable to sit in mid-line; is always falling over or leaning on supports;
- Excessively avoids, or alternately craves vestibular stimulation e.g. swinging, spinning, rocking, running, jumping;
- Avoids "looking up" or standing on one foot;
- Energy either zoned out and sleepy, or alternatively charged and hyper.

How to Ensure Adequate Vestibular Stimulation

The basic principles for vestibular stimulation in home, school and playground environments, is for children to engage in types of play or equipment that take them off their center of gravity. This challenges them to use their core stabilizer muscles to bring them back to center. Following are some examples of activities and equipment to stimulate a child's vestibular system, in home, school and community playground environments.

Activities: bike riding, swinging, jumping, spinning, tree climbing, rough and tumble play, wrestling, tag and other outdoor or gym games, gymnastics, swimming, jumping jacks.

Equipment:
- *Swings*: platform, tire, rope, traditional, frog, inner tube, glider;
- *Slides:* straight, circular, stepped;
- *Trampolines:* large give increase vestibular stimuli, small should have handle to hold onto;
- Merry-go-rounds, spinning discs, sit and spins, wobble boards;
- Therapy balls, move-n-sit cushions.

Chapter 14

The Proprioceptive System

My son sits on my lap so hard, and with so much force that it sometimes hurts! He is always accidentally hurting other children, as he doesn't seem to know the force he exerts during play. He is always pulling on my arm, or pushing me from behind, like he wants me to move faster, but we have no where to go!

From the moment my daughter started to move, it seemed as if she wanted to climb. She was climbing out of her car seat, play pen and crib when she was only 6 months old! Now she hangs on door frames, likes to move the fridge around the kitchen, and is always pushing, pulling, lifting and carrying things. She moves constantly, and never seems to settle down and rest. She is exhausting!

These are comments that are familiar with parents of children who have difficulty processing and integrating proprioceptive sensory stimuli. These children often "seek" proprioceptive, also termed "prop", stimulation to their joints and muscles to blow off some of their excess energy. Due to chronically high energy states, children who have proprioceptive sensory processing difficulties often get into a lot of trouble when they enter the daycare and preschool systems, as they are not aware of hurting their peers in what they would consider is normal play behavior.

Where is the Proprioceptive System Located?

The proprioceptive sensory system is located in the muscles and joints and is responsible for refined fine and gross motor movements necessary for printing, reading and sports. Children register proprioceptive stimuli through engaging in "heavy work" type activities involving resistive movements that load the joints and muscles. Participation in resistive activities would involve movements of either push, pull, lift or carry such as push ups, chin up bars, lifting bum off chair surface, or carrying bags of groceries or other heavy items.

The Proprioceptive System

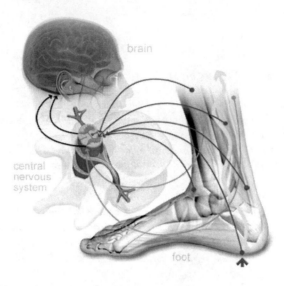

What is the Function of the Proprioceptive System?

The proprioceptive system works closely in conjunction with the tactile and vestibular sensory systems to allow a child to achieve a "sensory foundation", or an ability to know where their body is in space. Children with difficulties processing proprioceptive sensory information often will be observed "seeking" this type of stimuli through pushing, pulling, lifting or carrying heavy objects. Sensory seeking works to "ground" a child's energy, thus helping that child to feel centered and in their body. Proprioceptive stimulation therefore can have a calming effect on a child, as well as improved performance in both fine and gross motor tasks.

The proprioceptive system develops when a child performs "heavy work," such as rolling over as an infant, pulling to a standing position as a toddler, or rough house or explorative play as a child. While recent development of devices and techniques (such as child restraint bucket-type seats) have markedly improved our children's safety, they have inadvertently played a part in contributing to the developmental delays that we are observing in today's children. For example, the *Back to Sleep Program* developed by health professionals as an intervention for *Sudden Infant Death Syndrome* has resulted in parents being afraid to place their children on their stomachs during the daytime. While it is imperative that parents follow the *Back To Sleep Program* guidelines while an infant is unattended, e.g. night time in a crib, infants do require extensive "tummy time" when they are up during the day under a parent's supervision. Tummy time causes a child to utilize their proprioceptive system as they push up off their tummies to look around and see their world. Tummy time also provides deep pressure stimuli to an infant's tactile or touch receptors located in their stomach and groin areas, necessary for attaining eventual praxis and motor planning. If an infant does not receive adequate amounts of tummy time, the proprioceptive and tactile systems miss a critical element in development.

Why Children Who Don't Engage in "Heavy Work" Can't Learn

A child who has difficulty processing proprioceptive sensory stimuli, often moves constantly, and will employ "momentum" and fast movement during activities to compensate for the inability to execute refined gross and fine motor movements. Children with proprioceptive sensory processing difficulties will often be observed running constantly, with their upper body leading their lower body, bumping into objects and people as they move quickly through their world. These children often like to engage in "crash and bump" techniques, to increase proprioceptive input to the muscles and joints, which helps them to calm their energized system and to determine their position in space. It's important to realize that these children are not actually "clumsy" but are rather seeking the type of sensory stimuli that they need in order to achieve competence in fine and gross motor tasks. Children with difficulty processing proprioceptive sensory input often are poor printers and print "dark" letters, as their poor position sense impedes their muscle's ability to "know" how to execute motor plans necessary for stroke, shape and letter production.

While well meaning parents often try to make their infants and toddlers lives easier and more stimulating by placing them close to toys, mobiles and television, this deprives them of what they need for optimal sensory and motor development. Children need to move, touch, and explore their environment, and when restrained from doing so, will result in delays to development. While we need to keep our children safe and happy, there are many other ways that a parent can promote proprioceptive stimulation, e.g. creating a game by placing a toy slightly out of their infants reach, not picking up a toddler when they take a non-harmful tumble but rather gently encourage the toddler to get up on their own, or not over do child-proofing of homes - for example leave the safety lock off the pots and pans cupboard to optimize a child's exploration.

As toddlers grow into children, rough play is essential for proper proprioceptive system development. Running, climbing, jumping, hanging, and swinging are all essential for proper motor system development. These aforementioned play tasks stimulate the muscles and the joints, providing an adequate "body map" for the child, and a "grounding" of their energy body.

How to Know if a Child has a Proprioceptive Processing Problem

Following is a list of some common traits of children with proprioceptive dysfunction that you can easily identify by watching children move about in their environment:

- Weak extremities or grip strength; tires easily;
- Frequently pushes or pulls on objects or people;
- Hits self, others or body slams self against a wall or floor;
- Rough, ungraded movements;
- Hurts others unintentionally;
- Difficulty managing anger.

How to Ensure Adequate Proprioceptive Stimulation

The basic principles for proprioceptive or "prop" stimulation in home, school and playground environments, is for children to engage in types of play or equipment that require push, pull, lift and carry movements. This challenges them to use their gross and fine motor muscles and enables them to refine or modulate movements. Following are some examples of activities and equipment to stimulate a child's proprioceptive system, in home, school and community playground environments. Schools may want to make daily tasks for children that are perceived as "jobs" involving prop stimulation.

Activities: tug of war, digging in the garden or sand box, wheelbarrow races, carpet square races, carrying two milk jugs full of sand, climbing, wrestling.

Equipment:

- *Climbing:* frames, cargo ropes, climbing ropes, slide ladders, climbing walls;
- *Pushing:* hand/desk/floor/wall pushes, hand "push off" with partner, clean windows;
- *Pulling:* hand pull, chin up bar, deflated bike inner tubes;
- *Lifting:* stationary weights, shovel snow, carrying wood, moving tables/chairs, helping friends move;
- *Carrying:* 2 one gallon milk jugs full of sand, groceries, garbage, milk crates loaded with books.

For infants, make sure they have lots of supervised tummy time, and learn to roll over and make movements by themselves, as opposed to having the parent make movement easy for them. For toddlers, it's important to create a safe environment for exploratory play where they're encouraged to get up themselves when they fall. I'm not suggesting to just stand there watching your infant or toddler struggle. Why not get down on the floor with them, and teach them how to get up, or get on the floor with your toddler and teach them how to crawl, or get on the stairs and teach them how to climb.

Parents often ask why children need to run around prior to bed. This is child who is seeking proprioceptive input in order to calm themselves in preparation for eventual sleep. Rather than letting a child run all over the house, a far more effective technique prior to bedtime, would be to make sure the child receives the necessary proprioceptive input through a "heavy work" type of play e.g. having the child climb up onto the parents shoulders, arm wrestling, floor wrestling, climbing up a suspended rope, swinging from trapeze, and doing chin ups using a chin up bar, will all work to ground a child's energy and create a calm state for sleep. Parents should not allow their child to watch television or play video games for one hour prior to sleep, as this type of input "wakes up" the part of the brain that needs to go to sleep, and negates any benefits received from previous proprioceptive input.

Children who overuse technology are sedentary, and sedentary children have poorly developed proprioceptive systems. These children's muscles are either weak and "floppy", or strong, but with poor refined control. Children who overuse technology need to balance "input" activity with heavy work type "output" activities, such as lifting weights or play wrestling to promote optimal development.

Touch

While there are literally hundreds of research studies showing the positive benefits of holding and touching children, we are rapidly moving toward a time of "touch deprivation" for both children and their parents. Readers may have watched a recent movie called "Babies" where the film producer Thomas Balmes spent the first year of life of newborn infants with families from four different cultures. As the producer moved from Mongolia to Africa to Japan and to the United States, he beautifully captured the profoundly different ways in which we raise our children. There is no speaking in this film, and hence, no judgment regarding the different manner in which these children were raised. What struck me as a trained sensory therapist was the *sensory rich* nature-based environments that both the Mongolian and African babies were exposed to. Through self exploration, and play with their siblings, peers and mothers, these babies tactile systems were constantly being stimulated.

This section will discuss why touch is so important for child development, and how different types of touch can facilitate relaxation and calmness, as well as improve a child's ability to move their bodies in a smooth and planned manner.

Chapter 15

The Tactile System

Where is the Tactile System Located?

Our skin is the most basic and easy to understand sensory system. Covering every square inch of our body, the human touch system is highly sensitive and therefore highly reactive to changes in our environment. The tactile receptors are located in the skin. Human skin has a number of different types of receptors that detect changes in pressure, temperature, pain, as well as different types of touch sensations. Collectively speaking these receptors are called tactile receptors and carry information to the brain regarding the quality or quantity of sensation, and then the brain interprets this "message" and decides how to respond. Skin is the largest organ in the human body and if stretched out completely, an adult's skin would encompass a 20' X 20' area. The tactile system is highly innervated, with approximately 70,000 tactile receptors per square inch (Montagu, 1972). Due to this high receptor density, the tactile system is highly sensitive and reacts to subtle changes in the quality and quantity of touch, as well as to changes in the surrounding environment.

Tactile Receptors

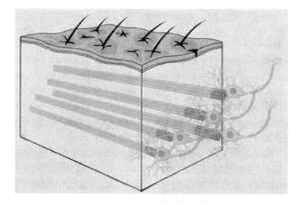

What is the Function of the Tactile System?

For over 50 years it has been documented in research literature that touch is not only a biological necessity, without which infants die, but touch has also been shown to improve overall sensory, motor and attachment development (Field, 1997). Acknowledgement of the tactile system as an integral organ of the human body came about through studies in the 1960's by a French physiologist professor Dr. Ashley Montagu who discovered that infant mortality could be markedly reduced through the simple intervention of human touch. Dr. Montagu was called to an orphanage to observe the ministrations of an elderly grandmother by the name of "Anna", who seemed to have the magic touch with low birth weight infants who had difficulty feeding, and hence were likely to not survive. Dr. Montagu observed Anna, who was a large, portly woman with "voluminous breasts", place babies "skin to skin" meaning that she bared her chest and placed the infant's skin in direct contact with her own skin. Although she was unable to nurse these babies, Anna provided another life sustaining gift, that of a loving, cooing voice, with warm and soft skin. As we can all guess, these babies that Anna cared for had significantly higher survival rates than those whom did not receive her wonderful care. And thus began the profound and world changing research by Dr. Montagu, who fostered a radical shift in infant care practices that are still with us today.

Dr. Montagu went on to write a monumental book titled *Touch: The Human Significance of the Skin*, where he documents numerous studies involving different types of touch with children. He found that children who receive adequate touch early in development were observed to be calm and relaxed, and children who receive inadequate touch appeared anxious and agitated. Pediatric researcher Ruth Feldman in 2002 performed a comparative study of two different types of neonatal infant care: the use of a "kangaroo care" where the infant was carried in a pouch-type device by the caregiver employing skin-to-skin contact, and the use of traditional incubators. Dr. Feldman found at 37 weeks gestational age, the kangaroo mothers showed more positive affect, touch, and adaptation to infant cues; and infants showed more alertness and less gaze aversion. Mothers reported less depression and perceived infants as less abnormal. Ann Bigelow, pediatric researcher at St. Francis Xavier University in Nova Scotia found that skin-to-skin tactile stimulation between mother and infant was shown to reduce gurgitation, improve sleep and overall growth, and enhance infants' sensitivity to their mother (Bigelow, 2006).

Why Children Who Are Not Touched Can't Learn

Dr. Jean Ayres, a leading researcher in the area of sensory integration, reports in her book *Sensory Integration and Learning Disorders,* that stimulation to the tactile system is integral for the formation of "praxis", or the ability to formulate motor plans for performing activities. Praxis is essential for children to be able to participate in sports, dress themselves, print, and even just walk across the room without bumping into things or falling over. Occupational therapy literature has reported tactile system dysfunction and praxis difficulties in children with a variety of disorders, including adhd and autism (May-Benson, 2007). In home settings, children can receive tactile stimulation through parental interactions such as hugs, book reading and snuggling, rough and tumble play with siblings and peers, and while at school through playground and gym play.

In clinic settings I have observed parents who demonstrate limited physical interactions with their children. They don't touch their child, and consequently this child appears to be suffering to some degree from parental "neglect". Children who are not touched have an *under developed* tactile system, and may demonstrate tactile sensitivities and/or "dyspraxia". These tactile sensitivities and dyspraxia affect a child's ability to plan and initiate movement, as well as result in a level of anxiety and agitation that limit attention and learning ability. Children with autism and adhd, as well as some children with learning disabilities, demonstrate tactile sensory system impairment. This dysfunction in the tactile system results in significant problems with self regulation affecting attention and learning ability, as well as problems with praxis affecting planning and initiating movement (Field, 1997; Lane, 2010; Parush, 2007). As a sensory therapist, whenever I observe limited child-parent interaction, facilitating parent-child connection is where I focus my initial intervention. Once the parent and child are more comfortable interacting in a play situation, the child receives improved input to their tactile system, enabling improved movement patterns. Failure to receive adequate touch through overuse of technology, also explains why technology is so damaging to a child's ability to learn. Extensive use of technology by parents and children has a direct effect of reducing the *amount* and *quality* of touch that parent and child give and receive, and contributes to resulting behaviors and "dyspraxia" characteristic with touch deprivation. Let me explain this concept of touch deprivation and dyspraxia further, as every parent, teacher and therapist should have a solid understanding of this concept in order to help these children.

Let's imagine for a moment a child who sees a toy across the room, and wants to go and pick it up. The first developmental component of *praxis*, is an "idea" in the child's brain about what it is they want to achieve e.g. picking up the toy. This is called *ideational praxis*. Many children with adhd and autism exhibit difficulty with ideational praxis, and run about "willy nilly", never seeming to engage in any activity. Technology overuse has caused extensive impairment in children's ability to create ideas of what they would like to do, and consequently, all children who overuse technology have some degree of *ideational praxis*.

Through prolonged exposure to technologies such as television, video games and internet, children view a two-dimensional image that has very little basis in three-dimensional relational reality. When these children turn the device off, they have limited previous experiences to reflect back upon or *remember,* in order to enable then to create an *idea* of what they would like to do. Termed "feedback loop", this lack of previous experience limits exploration and trial of new experiences. Many children have difficulty developing these *ideas* regarding tasks, and require this continuous feedback loop to show them in their "mind's eye" the task over and over again. This continuous feedback loop allows the child to then able to *execute* the movement. Children who overuse technology have a "poverty" of ideas and limited feedback loops, with consequent difficulty *executing* movements. Once an idea is formulated, children need to be able to send a message to their muscles to start them moving in the right direction. Once this movement is started, the tactile system provides feedback to the brain regarding foot placement on the floor and the sensation of air (and clothes), moving along the skin - giving the child a sense of movement through space. Children "feel" what it's like to do a task through their tactile system, and therefore adequate tactile systems allow children to learn how to plan and execute motor movements.

The final stage in praxis is to be able to *complete* movements. When execution is performed over and over, the task becomes ingrained into subconscious memory, a feedback loop is established, and the movement is developed into a proficient motor plan, allowing a child to *complete* the movement. How many times have parents, teachers and therapists struggled trying to teach a child a movement pattern, only to watch them repeated fail in their attempts. Using touch, in the form of hugs, weighted bean bags, or deep pressure touch techniques, can be very effective in helping a child to plan and execute movement. For parents and teachers to be able to fully understand and identify with a child who has tactile deprivation and difficulty with praxis, remember your previous task of writing your name mirror image backwards. The frustration and despair resulting from this experience is what it's like for many of our children who have praxis and motor planning difficulties. A connection statement such as "I see you are having difficulty", followed by a nice shoulder or hand squeeze, and then a lap or shoulder bean bag, can be very effective in promoting planned movement. The child may also benefit from "hands on" guidance through the movement pattern, but first the child should receive some connection and deep tactile pressure to calm their sensitive tactile system.

The tactile system develops very rapidly during early infant and toddler development, and therefore many factors can affect its development. We've known for many years that in vitro exposure to drugs and alcohol can create a tactile defensive child, requiring early intervention by occupational therapists in the area of tactile desensitization. We also know that children with some types of learning disabilities also have tactile sensory system impairment (May-Benson, 2007). These tactile problems cause a whole host of problems during a child's early years, but most pronounced when that child reaches school age. Children with tactile impairment often demonstrate symptoms of fright, flight or fight when exposed to "unexpected" touch - an often confusing response for parents to teachers. These children don't tolerate labels in clothing or anything tight-fitting, and prefer loose socks and pants. Tactile sensitive children also hate to have their teeth brushed or their hair combed. They also tend to be very picky eaters, with what can appear to be rather contradictory requests: e.g. preferring either bland foods in the "white" group, but also liking spicy salsa.

Technology Overuse Causes Touch Deprivation

Any time spent using technology is detrimental to child development, and gravely limits tactile input from siblings, parents, classmates and teachers. Instead of rocking our babies to sleep, we are putting televisions in their bedrooms. Instead of rough and tumble play with our toddlers before bed, we are letting them play video games with their older siblings, and then wonder why they can't get to sleep. Instead of reading to our pre-schooler before bed, we sit on the couch with them and watch a reality TV show. Instead of playing baseball in the back yard with our school-aged child, we buy him the latest new video game to buy us some time to be alone. In all of these scenarios, these children are not receiving life sustaining and comforting touch and human connection, and the outcomes will be problematic behaviors at home and at school.

Generally speaking, we are an advanced generation of well informed adults regarding what infants need to thrive and grow. We advocate for breast feeding and infant swaddling, although this doesn't always happen. In my private practice, I have seen a number of children with mal-developed tactile sensory systems who were premature births and were never breast fed or swaddled, despite the extensive research supporting the profound benefits of these techniques. There seems to be a new movement underway of parents who simply don't have the time to breast feed or practice swaddling or skin to skin touch, and are consequently reverting to the use of bottles, bucket seats and televisions to pacify their upset infant.

This lack of tactile input is resulting in screaming and outraged babies who know what they need, and are not getting it. As discussed further in future chapters covering attachment theory, these babies learn to either cry longer and harder to get that life sustaining touch, or they simply give up and repress their needs, hoping Mom or Dad will take notice and care for them if they are quiet. Either response to the lack of touch and human connection, will result in a child with dysfunctional yet adaptive coping strategies to get their needs met. These strategies are usually described as "difficult behaviors" by the health and education systems, and are likely to result in these children getting themselves diagnosed with some form of new age mental illness and medication.

How to Know if s Child has a Tactile Processing Problem

We need to help these children with tactile processing dysfunction discover that the skin that they've been encased in for however many years, is actually theirs! Many children with touch system impairment explain that they don't feel like their skin is their "own". They describe that they feel as if bees are biting them, or they've got a million mosquito bites that they can't scratch. Women might relate to these tactile disturbances as akin to trying to break in a new bra with a very firm under-wire, or for men wearing a pair of underwear that is far too tight and pants that are cutting everywhere that you don't want them too. Following this case scenario, by the end of the day any adult would be frustrated, agitated and generally miserable. Fortunately as adults we can remove these garments, but these children can't remove their skin. Following is a list of some common traits of children with tactile dysfunction that you can easily identify by watching how children react to touch in their environment:

- Reacts negatively to unexpected touch
- Hates clothing labels or scratchy clothing; dislikes hair or teeth brushing
- Picky about different textured (as opposed to tastes) of foods
- Likes one texture of noodle, and not another
- Touches everything, but doesn't like to be touched by others
- Loves deep pressure hugs
- Highly agitated and anxious

How to Ensure Adequate Tactile Stimulation

The basic principles for tactile stimulation in home, school and playground environments, is for children to engage in types of play or equipment that involve "predictable" deep pressure to the skin, preferably initiated on their own. This allows the child a sense of control over their seemingly uncontrollable environment, and serves to reduce cortisol and adrenalin levels, thus inducing a calming experience. Following are some examples of activities and equipment to stimulate a child's tactile system, in home, school and community playground environments.

Deep Pressure Touch Activities

- *Shoulder Squeeze*

Deep Pressure Touch (DPT) techniques involve firm sustained pressure to the skin, either through skin to skin touch, or use of a device. A useful DPT technique is the "shoulder squeeze". This technique involves placing your hands firmly on the child's shoulders with the outside arm pressed firmly on the child's upper back and creating and "in and down" pressure. As with any sensory strategy, it is very important for the teacher or parent to follow outlined procedures, as described below:

1. Offer the child some *connection* by saying an "I see" or "I hear" statements such as "I see you are getting upset;
2. Ask the child for permission: "Would you like a shoulder squeeze?" If the child says "Yes"...;
3. Approach the child from the front, so that they can see what you are doing, and stand off to the side with your body positioned as far away as possible from their body, both looking in the same direction;
4. Place your hands one on each shoulder, and your arm firmly across the child's back and initiate a firm squeeze of the shoulders in an inward and downward motion;
5. Ask the child how they are doing, and look for an *adaptive* or positive response. Should the child move away from you, stop immediately;
6. Sustain DPT technique until the child wants you to stop; generally about 1-2 minutes duration.

Caution: Be sure your body is as far away from the child as possible, in order to ensure that DPT is not mistakenly interpreted as a form of "sexual touch" by other teachers, parents or the student themselves. Some other DPT techniques are as follows:

- *Steamroller:* have the child lie on their stomach and roll a therapy ball firmly over the backs of their feet, legs, and back (not neck or head);
- *Sandwich:* squeeze the child between two beanbag chairs, or have the child lie between the couch base and the cushions, or the box spring and a mattress and place firm pressure on the child's skin. Ensure no equipment is placed over the child's face;
- *Burrito:* wrap the child tightly in a blanket followed by firmly rubbing whatever

"sauce" the child requests onto their arms and legs;
- *Huggie chair:* get a sweat shirt or sports jersey, and sew together the neck pieces, and a line between both armpits, effectively creating a "tube" to pack arms and neck with bags of lentils or rice. Place this shirt over the back of a chair. Children can sit in the chair and wrap the arms around their neck and cross over their chest, effectively giving themselves a hug.

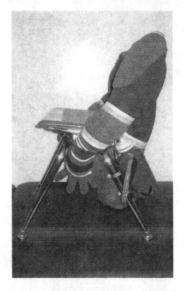

All of these techniques are to be done with the child's permission, as well as continually monitoring the child for an adaptive response indicating that the child finds these techniques pleasurable. At no time should these techniques ever be initiated on a child who resists them, since to be effective, the child should ask for and enjoy them! A child who resists these techniques likely requires referral to an occupational therapist trained in sensory integration therapy for further assessment and specific interventions.

Equipment:

- Lycra pod swing
- 3 truck tire inner tubes tied together; crawl inside
- Pod type net swings
- Body pillows around child at night in bed, or in chair during day
- Bean bag chairs
- Tent full of pillows and blankets in classroom
- Weighted neck tubes or lap bags

Now that readers understand how to stimulate a child's vestibular, proprioceptive and tactile sensory systems, types of activities and equipment are endless. Please refer to *Zone'in Recommended Tools and Techniques* at the end of this section for more ideas. Remember, children cannot get vestibular, proprioceptive or tactile stimulation from technology, so cover up those televisions and computers with a blanket, or store them away, and have some fun!

Zone'in Recommended Tools

Zone'in Tools	Sensory System	Desired Outcome	Supplier
Require $ Purchase			
Zone'in Program	All of them!	Improved attention	www.zonein.ca
Metronome	Auditory/Vestibular	Fluidity of movement	Music outlets
Rhythmic Entrainment Intervention	Auditory	Calming	www.REIinstitute.com
Journey to the Wild Devine videogame; D. Chopra	Parasympathetic Nervous System, Vagus	Calming	www.chopra.com
The Journey for Kids	Cellular healing	calming	www.thejourney.com
The Flow (water tube)	Vestibular - bilateral coordination, postural tone	Fluidity for reading and printing	www.pdppro.com
Colored Therapy Glasses	Visual	Reduced visual sensitivity	www.toolsforwellness.com
"Z" Vibe	Oral	Alerting	www.therapyshoppe.com
The Cardio Blade Wobble Board	Vestibular – bilateral coordination, postural tone	Core stability; fluidity for reading and printing	www.fitter1.com
Platform Swing	Vestibular stimulation	Posture and coordination improvement, optimal arousal state	www.southpawenterprises.com
Jump Rope	Vestibular, rhythm	Alerting	Canadian Tire, Walmart
Lycra Pod Swing	Tactile – deep pressure	Calming	www.schoolspecialityonline.com
Weighted Devices	Tactile – deep pressure	Calming	www.innovaid.ca
Therapy Ball	Vestibular – postural tone Tactile – deep pressure	Calming	Canadian Tire, Walmart, therapy outlets
Gym Spin Disc – or - Dizzy Disc	Vestibular	Alerting	www.sensoryseekers.com
Caterpillar tube	Tactile/Visual/Motor planning	Calming, praxis	www.schoolspecialityonline.com
Tent with Pillows	Visual and Auditory	Calming	Ikea or Sears
Ear Plugs or iPods	Auditory Filter	Improved attention for desk work	Create *Zone'in Tool Rules* of use only while teacher isn't talking
Free!			
Used Bike Inner Tubes – Deflated	Proprioceptive	Calming/Alerting	Local bike store
Used Truck Inner Tubes – Inflated	Tactile – deep pressure	Calming	Local tire store
Duvet Cover with Lots of Foam Chips – Crash and Bump Technique	Tactile – deep pressure Proprioceptive, Vestibular	Calming	Local foam store, garage sales
Mini - Tramps	Vestibular	Calming/Alerting	Garage sales, Sears
Old Exercise Bikes – High Resistance	Proprioceptive	Calming	Garage sales, parent's basements
Carpet Squares	Tact/Vestib/Prop	In the Zone!	Carpet suppliers
Chin Up Bars	Proprioceptive	Calming	Garage sales, Canadian Tire
Huggie Chair	Tactile – Deep Pressure	Calming	Hockey shirt, bean bags, chair
Rocking Chair	Vestibular	Calming	Garage sale, parent's

Zone'in Recommended Techniques

Zone'in Techniques	Sensory System	Desired Outcome	Method
30 Seconds No Movement	Energy baseline	Insight	Reduce visual clutter, no movement 30 seconds
Infinity Walk	Vestibular, proprioceptive and visual systems	Improve posture, coordination and arousal states.	Walk in an infinity around 2 obstacles while reading flash cards.
Infinity Eye Movement	Vestibular and visual systems	Improves oculomotor coordination for printing and reading	Eyes trace large infinity pattern drawn on board.
Infinity Draw	Vestibular, visual and fine motor	Improves fine motor coordination for printing	Draw infinity pattern on board or at desk
Hand/Shoulder/Chair/Desk/Wall - Push/Pull	Proprioceptive and tactile systems	Optimal arousal	Push hard for count of 10, followed by deep breath.
Three Deep Breaths	Parasympathetic Nervous System	Calming	Each time breathe in/out, force residual volume.
Square Breathing	Vestibular and neck proprioceptive systems	Alerting	Fixate upper left corner of wall, inhale across, exhale down, inhale back, exhale up.
The Tree	Proprioceptive and parasympathetic NS	Calming	Trunk strong and tall, roots rooted, branches/leaves reaching the sun.
The Breath Push	Proprioceptive and parasympathetic NS	Blowing off carbon dioxide build-up; good for ADHD	Wrist back, palm open, like saying "Stop"!
Ear Rub	Auditory and tactile systems	Improved auditory comprehension	Vigorously rub outer borders of ears and lobes.
Ear Cupping	Auditory	Improved auditory comprehension	Student cups hands over ears – open to teacher
Shoulder Squeeze	Tactile/Proprioceptive and Attachment	Calming	Ask permission, stand to side of student, one arm across back , hands on shoulders, squeeze "in and down" motion for ~ 60 seconds
Hand Hold/Eye Contact	Tactile/Attachment	Calming	Use "I see..." statements e.g. "I see you are struggling with your math"
Bum Walking	Vestibular, proprioceptive, and tactile systems	Bilateral integration, postural tone	Sitting on floor, legs extended, elbows bent, walk bum across floor
Crab Walk/Wheelbarrow	Proprioceptive!!! and vestibular systems	Postural tone, bilateral integration, arm and leg strengthening	Crab walk: tummy down or up Wheelbarrow: one's the wheel, other the barrow
Super(wo)man!	Back and neck extension	Postural tone	Lye on floor on tummy, lift legs, arms and head off floor
The Cat	Back and neck extension	Postural tone	Four point kneeling, arch/slump back
Crash and Bump	Proprioception	Alerting and calming	Run and jump into pile of pillows
Motor Mountains	Visual motor	Preparatory for printing	Drive car or pen over mountains drawn on butcher paper
Add your own Zone'in Techniques!			

Additional Sensory Resources

The following two DVD's are great resources for parents, teachers and therapists regarding sensory processing and strategies:

- *A Sensory World: Making Sense of Sensory Disorders* by TCU Institute of Child Development. This DVD offers examples of combining vestibular, proprioceptive, tactile and attachment techniques in a variety of settings.

- *Applying Sensory Integration Principles Where Children Live, Learn and Play* by Pediatric Therapy Network. This DVD describes sensory integration principles, as well as application in home, classroom, clinic and community settings.

Views of a Pediatric Occupational Therapist

Today there is a lot of visual and auditory information and less tactile, vestibular and proprioceptive information. For that reason kids are less balanced and lack motor abilities, resulting in behavior and motor problems. In the Netherlands in today's paper there was an issue on fall-training in schools, because last year there was an increase of falling in kids, which causes a lot more fractures. This is produced by kids being less able in motor activities, and increased in weight, both caused by not moving enough.

Kids need being touched, being moved and space to move and play by them self. In this way they would be involved in the activities they do, and not occupied too much with virtual games. Kids need to explore their own possibilities without adults telling them too much what to do and what not to do.

Only by doing, do kids get necessary proprioceptive information about the success of their activities, this proprioceptive feedback is not only important for learning motor skills but a necessity for concentration. Proprioceptive sensory information keeps them balanced and focused on the tasks they are doing; only then can they can start to integrate visual and auditory information as well.

Proprioceptive sensory information is the main key to reduce sensory processing disorder. This is the main reason why I set up a website with simple games to do for parents with their virtual kids.

Els Rengenhart, Occupational Therapist, sensoryprocessing.info

Connection

Readers may have watched a recent movie called "Surrogate" where humans lye on their beds at home 24/7 electronically "plugged" into their surrogate body, which is a robotic type device. The surrogate lives outside in the real world, while the human stays home in bed. Humans can pick out their own surrogate, just like they'd pick out a new dress. Of course, the surrogate never get sick or injured, in fact they are just about perfect in every way. The humans interact through the interface of the surrogate body, so while the human wife might be lying in a bed in the next room, the husband would be interacting with her "physically" through her surrogate, which could be anywhere outside – work, gym, or the bar. The humans are all on "polypharmacy" and taking a significant amount of medication, and look like, well, not too good. While the premise of this movie might seem far-fetched at first, upon further consideration, we are almost already there. We already have numerous devices that act as an interface between humans. Whether it is email, texting, or Facebook, new age technologies are forever changing the ways in which we relate (or not) as human beings.

This section will discuss why human connection is so important for child mental health and social ability, and how the child becomes affected when attachment formation is less than optimal.

Chapter 16

Attachment – Engaging the Outside World

I've completed a number of courses on attachment theory and treatment over the past three years, predominantly following the work of Kim Barthel, Occupational Therapist and Dr. Pat Crittenden who developed the *Dynamic Maturational Model of Attachment* and authored the book *Raising Parents: Attachment, Parenting and Child Safety*. Information gleaned from these courses raises considerable concern regarding the propensity of the 21st century to detach from reality and attach to devices. The permeation of technology into home and school-based settings, has resulted in technology becoming an "interface" between adults and children. Connection to technology is disconnecting human relationship at a rapid pace, with far reaching and devastating consequences for our children. Quite frankly, many adults do not know *how* to relate with each other anymore in a meaningful manner, much less do they know how to relate to children. This is causing a deepening and widening chasm between adults and children, a chasm that soon will be too wide to bridge the gap and repair.

Human attachment is a *biological need*, without which we would die. For hundreds of years, human beings have been "pack" animals, with an established intrinsic role and purpose. While technology was designed for human efficiency, it has also has the effect of distancing humans from each other and diminishing the need for the human "pack". Can human beings adapt to this growing sense of isolation from each other, and what will be the impact on young infants and children who have little or no intimate contact with their parents? This section will provide readers with a brief review of attachment theory, and application of attachment theory to current technology usage, both with parents and teachers.

The quality and quantity of time that a parent spends with their child has significant impact on many aspects of the child's mental health and well being. Human connection or attachment theory first originated with the work of John Bowlby and Mary Ainsworth, British psychoanalysts who reported that the primary "job" of the developing infant is to form a life sustaining attachment with their primary caregiver (Bowlby, 1990). Bowlby and Ainsworth state that without this primary attachment bonding, the infant will not survive. It is generally reported in the research literature that the critical period for primary attachment formation is the first year of an infant's life; however some researchers state that in the case of dysfunctional or even failed attachment formation, primary attachments can be established throughout childhood and even into adulthood (Crittenden, 2008; Welch, 2008).

Attachment Theory

Attachment is, in its simplest form, about human survival. Bowlby identified that every infant, toddler and child require a "secure base" from which they can move out into the world, and a "safe haven" where they can return to organize themselves. Bowlby defined attachment as an emotional bond between parent and child, essential for survival as the attachment bond allows the child to get their survival needs met. While the job of the infant is to attach to the parent, the job of the parent regarding facilitating healthy attachment is two-fold: to provide this "safe haven" for the child to return to when stressed, and to "launch" the child into the world for self-exploration. Although attachment theory varies slightly with different researchers, it is generally agreed that there are four types of attachment behavior patterns that stem from failure of the parent to facilitate healthy attachment.

Type A – *Avoidant attachment*: the parent rejects, neglects, abuses or ridicules the child. Type A children minimize their emotions when distressed and *repress* their feelings, becoming overly reliant on them *self* to get their needs met. Type A children recognize the parent's need to *not* be needed.

Type B – *Secure attachment*: the parent is consistent and predictable with the child, and the child learns they can get their needs met simply by expressing their desires.

Type C – *Ambivalent attachment*: the parent is unpredictable and inconsistent with the child, but eventually if the child makes enough of a fuss, the parent will see to their needs. Type C children show extreme negative emotion when distressed, excessively *express* their feelings, and become overly reliant on others to get their needs met.

Type D – *Disorganized attachment*: the parent fluctuates between avoidant and ambivalent types of attachment behavior such as is found in parents with drug and/or alcohol addictions. The result is that the parent never truly meets the needs of the child. Type D children usually experience significant abuse or neglect, and suffer extreme forms of mental illness or eventual incarceration.

Attachment Formation and Parent Technology Use

To the best of my knowledge, the impact of technology on primary attachment formation has unfortunately not received the attention of the research community. Existing addiction research indicates that fear of intimacy is an underlying factor for addictions in adults, and this fear has it's origin in failed primary attachment (Flores, 2004). We also know that attachment to technologies such as televisions, movies, internet, video games, cell phones and iPods are resulting in a "detachment" from all that is human. Human detachment resulting from technology overuse is happening at such a rapid pace, it's difficult to determine what would be the immediate, much less the long term effects. One only has to reflect on current child health and academic statistics to know that something is seriously wrong with how we are raising and schooling our children.

With all this connection to technology, primary relationships are disconnecting, or worse, not even forming at all. Human attachment profoundly influences every aspect of human development: mind, body, emotions, social ability, values and productivity. We know that securely attached infants, toddlers and children have better self esteem, independence, autonomy, enduring friendships, trust and intimacy, impulse control, empathy and compassion, and resilience. What will happen when Type A and C attachment styles dominate society? What will Type A and C parents be like, and what type of third generation detached children will they produce? Relatedness will truly be a character trait of the past, as human beings grow ever more isolated, yet at the same time, ever more needy.

We all do it. We all, at some time or another, prefer to pick up the remote or Blackberry, or connect to the internet or television – rather than have a conversation with our spouse, children or co-workers. Sometimes connecting to the virtual world is just easier than connecting to humans, and at first glance, appears to be a lot more interesting and exciting. Let's face it, for years human relationships have proven to be complex, confusing, and down right difficult, resulting in a myriad of self help books, therapies, foster children (resulting from abuse or neglect), and divorce. What is unique about human relationships in the 21st century, is that the performance bar has now been set higher. To get a little bit of love and human connection, parents, children and workers are now required to compete with the seductive lure of technology, which is threatening the very fabric of life as we know it. While change and technological advancement can have a positive impact on society, if it is unmanaged and unregulated, the results can be devastating.

Four Way Disconnect

Human beings are now on the verge of what can be termed the "Four Way Disconnect" – from *self, others, nature* and *spirit*. Identity and attachment formation can only happen in relationship to others, and is best facilitated in nature based settings. Connection to technology is causing a disconnection from what we used to hold dear and close to our hearts, our children. Based on the ways in which the parent copes with the stresses of their own technology overuse, the parent, might raise their child in such a way as to result in either an avoidant, ambivalent, or disorganized attachment disorder. A study conducted in Beijing, China reports that adolescents with internet addictions consistently rated parental rearing behaviors as being over-intrusive, punitive, and lacking in responsiveness, indicating that the influences of parenting style and family function are important factors in the development of internet dependency (Xiuquin, 2010). Phillip Flores, a psychologist and author of the book 2004 *Addiction as an Attachment Disorder*, supports the theory that the underlying causal factor for addictions are malformed attachments with a primary parent, and that the way to treat addictions, is by treating the attachment disorder. Attachment disorders in children may be misdiagnosed as problem behaviors, mental illness, or be contributing factors to learning difficulties. As stated previously, a commonality between autism and adhd is that they are both considered to be attachment disorders (Mate, 2007; Mukaddes, 2000). Technology despite all its advantages is resulting in the human four way disconnect from *self, others, nature* and *spirit*. As the incidence of technology addictions continue to escalate in both parents and children, identifying and treating underlying attachment disorders will be the challenge of many health and education professionals for years to come.

Attachment Techniques

There are many different types of theories on attachment and just as many types of attachment building techniques. I will be restricting my comments and suggestions to the most basic and simple strategies. I strongly recommend that parents who have been unsuccessful in forming healthy attachments with their children, seek the assistance of an occupational therapist, counselor, psychologist or psychiatrist who is trained in attachment theory. For example, if a parent suffered a post-partum depression, marital breakdown, or death of a family member during the first year of their child's life, they may not have provided their child with the connection they needed to establish a healthy attachment base. With professional help and support, this attachment bond can still be formed with either the primary parent, or with close friends and/or family. Is the child healthy, happy and well adjusted? Then don't worry. If the infant, toddler or child cries excessively, has what appears to be an excess of temper tantrums, or is withdrawn and non-communicative, these may be signs that this child could benefit from the services of an expert in attachment assessment and treatment.

I have created an *Attachment Questionnaire* that will help parents to discover what areas they might improve on regarding their relationship with their child. These questions are designed to also offer ideas for attachment forming techniques. Every child wants to know that their parent is there for them. This "presence" can be communicated either verbally with "I see you" or "I hear you" statements, or non-verbally through hugs or pats on the back. Being a single parent with my first child, I always found that coming home from a long day at work was most difficult the first few minutes we walked through the door. My son had not seen me all day and was missing me, and I had been engrossed in some crisis or another at work and really just needed some "down" time. I used to start right into the making dinner routine, with my son at my feet demanding my attention in one way or another. This routine never worked for either of us, and sometimes would escalate into me getting angry and my son getting upset. I quickly found that if we both just made a cup of "kid tea" (loads of milk and honey) and sat down and read a book together, within minutes we were both relaxed and laughing and quite ready to start our evening time together on the right foot.

Attachment Questionnaire

		Yes	No
1.	**Past Parental Relationships**: "Although my parents may have worked or been quite busy, I knew I was loved and cared for most of the time by one or both of my parents."		
2.	**Intimacy Comfort Level**: "I feel comfortable showing intimacy with my children either through touch or words."		
3.	**Demonstrative - Touch**: "I touch my children at least once per day in a show of affection" (parents – hugs, teachers – hand touch to shoulder/arm). - or- **Demonstrative - Verbal**: "On a daily basis, I tell my children one positive attribute about themselves to build their self esteem."		
4.	**Available**: "I make myself available to interact with my children on a regular, scheduled daily basis" e.g. meals or recess.		
5.	**Responsive**: "When asked a question by my children, I generally stop what I'm doing, make eye contact, and answer the question as best I can."		
6.	**Receptive**: "When my child has something to tell me, I listen and ask questions, before I react to what they are saying."		
7.	**Interactive**: "Rather than "preach" to my children, I encourage questions and healthy interaction of thoughts and ideas."		
8.	**Attached**: "I know my children feel loved and cared for most of the time by me."		

Total number of "yes" answers _____

If you answered "yes" to all eight questions congratulations, you are a wonderful parent or teacher. If you answered "yes" to less than eight questions, you are still likely a wonderful parent or teacher, but I also hope this questionnaire has pointed out some areas that you can work on to improve your attachment and connection with your children.

Personal Attachment Plan

I, _____plan to increase the amount of time spent with my children performing activities other than watching television, in order to improve attachment and connection, from my current _____ minutes/hours per day up to _____ minutes/hours per day.

Instead of using television, cell phones, video games or internet, I plan to do the following attachment and connection building activities with my children (circle or add new ones): reading them a book every night, family wrestling night, dancing, biking, climbing trees, playing sports, baking, sewing, playing cards and/or board games, playing outdoor games, do volunteer work, visit elderly people, garden, do family chores, build something, take something apart, or...........

_____

_____

Generational Healing

Parents who have difficulty forming relationships with their children, likely had difficult relationships with their own parents. It is imperative for professionals to realize that many parents simply don't know how to form meaningful connections with their children, because they were never parented properly themselves. Parents who are unable to form healthy attachments with their children likely have limited knowledge about healthy relationship forming, as this was not their experience with their own parent.

On numerous occasions I have sat with parents and their child, and taught them how to "hold space" or be fully present and attentive with their child. This is a first stage in attachment formation. If a parent cannot be present and open for connection and attachment, it will never happen. During this time of holding space, the parent doesn't need to do anything, just be available to the child and non-reactive if the child is upset. The next stage is for the parent to offer positive affirmations to the child, or tell the child how much they love them. It is absolutely imperative that these positive comments be authentic and realistic, as connections and attachments do not form in the presence of inflated truths or outright lies. Therapists can teach parents how to hold their children, how to create that "secure base", and also teach them how to "launch" their child from this secure base. Parents who did not have healthy attachments with their own parents can overcome these obstacles to form meaningful relationships with their own children. They just need to be taught how.

Termed "Generational Healing", parents healing relationships with their own parents, will vastly improve relationships with their own children.

In the third section of *Virtual Child*, I will be offering parents a variety of *Balanced Technology Management* initiatives that will all work toward building the attachment system. It's never too late to form connections with your children, no matter how old they are.

Chapter 17

Addictions – Failure of the Attachment System

Media and society in general exhibit a "selective blindness" regarding the epidemic of childhood television, video game, internet and cell phone addictions. Technology addictions are the most socially acceptable form of addiction, which is why so few professionals will admit to its presence. While numerous research studies have reported causal links between technology use and a multitude of physical, mental, social and academic disorders, the media rarely reports these studies, and when they do, parents and teachers appear not to listen. Why is this? In numerous meeting and workshop environments, I've relayed to parents the perils of technology use with frequent responses of "Well, my child only watches the nature or the history channels", or "My child just uses the internet for their homework." During these discussions, I often observe parents with the "blank stare" look on their faces, as they dispute current research with disbelief and state comments like "My children can't possibly be watching *that* much television, when would they have time do anything else?" while never admitting their children doesn't do anything but technology.

Touch and Attachment Formation

Connection is an energetic form of attachment, a primary bond that begins in the womb, and is an essential force without which we would die. We learned earlier that touch is also a life sustaining need. As a result of recent advances in technology, we are once again are reverting back to live in a *touch deprived* world. Touch is an essential life force. As important as breathing is to the *physical* body, touch is to the *feeling* body. Touch and human connection, termed "attachment" are both essential ingredients for adequate child development, and form the foundation for eventual attention and learning ability.

In his 2007 book *Neurobehavioural Social Emotional Development in Infants*, Dr. Ed Tronick, Associate Professor of Pediatrics and Psychiatry, and Director of the *Boston Children's Hospital Child Development Unit,* reports that studies show that the infant sleep state is a "co-regulated process between the parent and infant, and is greatly affected by the quality and timing of the parental caretaking." Dr. Tronick reports that sleep/wake cycles are *innate,* and that the infant is born with their own pattern of *sleep rhythmicity*. He therefore opposes "fixed schedule" feeding and sleeping routines, and is a proponent of what he terms baby initiated "state contingent" patterning, which is the parent responding to the baby's needs. How well a parent is able to determine exactly what an infant needs, and then meet those needs immediately and effectively, results in a baby who is able to predict their environment and trust their parent to meet their needs. A parent who sets a schedule and/or routine that meets the *parent's* needs and not those of the infant, erodes the fragile parent-infant attachment formation. Failure to form a predictable attachment base, even in the first few weeks of an infant's life, will result in the baby "disconnecting" from the parent as a possible attachment figure. Letting these babies "cry it out" while the parent is busy doing their emails, surfing the net, or watching television, will result in *increased* crying in infants, and eventual tantrums and severe behavior issues when that infant grows to become a toddler.

As a society, we have confused what it means to be concerned with the well being and nourishment of our children, with what it means to give love and affection. Dr. Montagu describes a study where he looked at the amount of physical contact a parent gave to their children as an infant, toddler and young child. Surprisingly, the time of greatest physical contact is when a child is a toddler, not an infant as one would have thought. This fact was explained in light of the safety interventions a parent is required to make in the "caregiver" role for their toddler, pointing out the now broad distinction between care giving and showing love and affection for children.

What happened to cuddling children at night, reading a book, playing a game? Now we watch television. We rarely touch our children anymore, and actually create devices that distance the parents from the child! In efforts to promote safety, well meaning parents are impairing essential attachment development by unknowingly isolating themselves from their infants by using infant car seats. These "bucket seats", while intended to be used in the car, are now being used everywhere, and are replacing the primary contact that infants require to their touch systems received from being carried by their parents. Infants as young as 2-3 months are being placed in front of televisions, encased in bucket seats, where even just ten years ago, babies were carried everywhere by mom or dad, in sling like devices which allowed close body contact and loads of touch and movement stimulation. Feeling the rhythms of their parent's bodies, young neurological systems learned a tremendous amount through the rich and varied stimulation to their touch and balance systems, stimulation that is vastly important for proper neurological and attachment development.

Addictions Don't Fall Far From the Tree

Busy parents today seem to have great difficulty dealing with any problems their children might have, not due to a lack of love or commitment, but apparently due to the fact that they are just too busy. Admitting that they themselves and/or their child has an addiction to television, video games, internet or texting, may just be "the straw that breaks the camel's back" so to speak, and tip parents over that precarious edge of keeping it all together. Studies have shown that the apple doesn't fall far from the tree when looking at television and video game addictions in parents and children. Mukkades found in a 2002 study that children with higher than average technology usage had parents with higher than average usage. Mukkades also found that children of parents with high television usage were more likely than children of parents with low television usage, to demonstrate symptoms of reactive attachment disorder characterized by a severely disturbed ability to relate in a social manner with others.

Mukkades goes on to report that children with reactive attachment disorder are frequently misdiagnosed with autism, and that these misdiagnosed children respond well to behavioral therapy and training - not for the children, but for the parents. Since autism is the second fastest rising childhood mental disorder diagnosis, second only to anxiety, it might be worthwhile expanding autism treatment to trials of television and video game reduction, accompanied by attachment training for the autistic child's parents. Dr. Martha Welch, child psychiatrist and author of the book *Holding Time*, reports a study where a therapist trained the primary caregiver (in most cases the mother) to hold her child with autism on her lap facing her, while the mother's partner put their arm around the mother. While the child with autism struggled at first, the child slowly grew comfortable with this arrangement and began to establish eye contact with the mother. Dr. Welch cautions that this treatment is not to be performed by anyone other than the child's primary parents assisted by an attachment therapist, as it is the primary bonding by child and parent that this treatment is designed to facilitate. Since all children with technology addictions likely have parents who are addicted as well, and the underlying causal factor for these addictions are failure of the primary attachment system, our job as professionals is to facilitate attachment bonding. Designing family technology addiction treatments and training education and health professionals in the area of addictions and attachment, is the way toward a sustainable future for our children.

How does a parent know if they or their child has a technology addiction? Quite simply, when the choice of plugging into some form of technology is no longer a "choice", then it has become an "addiction". When someone feels compelled to grab the remote, as opposed to have a conversation with their child or partner, then this person might want to look at the fact that they may have an addiction. Consider the origin of addictions, whether it be to alcohol, drugs, gambling, or pornography. Hofler and Kooyman in a 1996 study reported that addiction actually has its origins in a fear of intimacy, and found that using a "therapeutic bonding" treatment protocol in adults improved their addiction status. Choosing to pick up the remote, cell phone, or doing emails after work hours, instead of connecting with children and partners, are all signs of addiction to technology, and greatly influence a parent's ability to connect in a significant way with their children. Addictions are prevalent in today's prevalent stressed out society, and unknowingly and unfortunately, these technology addicted adults are acting as primary role models to their highly impressionable children.

Section Summary

I've discussed in Section II that the three critical factors for the developing child, are to move, touch and be touched, and develop healthy attachments through the experience of human connection. The absence of these three critical factors for development, such as is caused by technology overuse, will cause devastating consequences to families and classrooms everywhere, and threaten the very sustainability of our children. I have developed a graphic titled *Critical Factors for Child Development* to summarize key concepts and show readers where we are heading when we choose to disconnect from humanity, and connect to a device. This graphic will guide readers toward the next and last section of *Virtual Child*, Section III on *Balanced Technology Management* initiatives through *Creating Sustainable Futures*. Let's look at what we all can do to reverse the detrimental effects of technology overuse on our children, and move them toward happy and healthy lives.

Critical Factors for Child Development

Critical Factors for Child Development

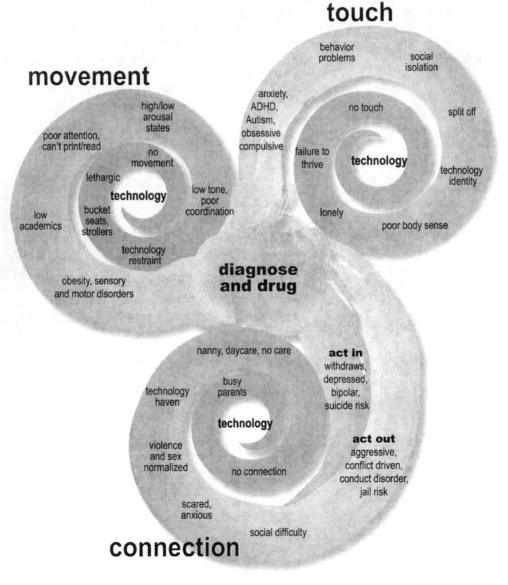

touch

behavior problems

social isolation

movement

anxiety, ADHD, Autism, obsessive compulsive

no touch

split off

high/low arousal states

poor attention, can't print/read

no movement

failure to thrive

technology

lethargic

technology identity

technology

low tone, poor coordination

low academics

bucket seats, strollers

lonely

poor body sense

technology restraint

obesity, sensory and motor disorders

diagnose and drug

nanny, daycare, no care

act in
withdraws, depressed, bipolar, suicide risk

technology haven

busy parents

technology

violence and sex normalized

no connection

act out
aggressive, conflict driven, conduct disorder, jail risk

scared, anxious

social difficulty

connection

© Zone'in Programs Inc. 2008

Chapter 18

Inner Drive – Building Skills and Confidence, in Areas Other Than Technology

A Professor in Child Development Speaks Out About the Impact of Technology on Play

In the end, a playful childhood is the most basic right of every child.

Free, self-initiated and spontaneous play is of utmost importance to a child's healthy mental, emotional and social development. This type of play is increasingly silenced by technology.

Electronic media has simply reinforced our need to hurry and our ability to get things done quickly. Much of this spills over into our child rearing and education. In many ways our new technologies have radically transformed childhood, and not always for the better.

David Elkind, Professor of Child Development at Tufts University and Author

What is Inner Drive?

Have you ever witnessed a child who just simply "lights up" when faced with an intriguing or challenging task? With a big smile and a twinkle in their eyes, these children are curious, creative, independent, and seem to tackle all their problems with desire and enthusiasm. They fall to bed each night physically exhausted, happy, and excited to wake up the next day to yet another challenge. This energetic state is what occupational therapists term "inner drive", a motivating force for children to engage in tasks and activities, without fear of failure. *Inner drive* "pushes" a child beyond their self perceived limitations, to be physically active, take on challenges, and ultimately get whatever it is they desire or think they need. Inner drive "drives" child development, and is an innate, motivating force for child survival.

Inner drive is what enables children to get out of bed in the morning, or go to bed at night without being told to. These children know what their body needs, and when they get their needs met, they feel good about themselves. Children with inner drive eat healthy food, know to take their vitamins, and make sure they get enough exercise and outdoor playtime. Readers are likely wondering who I'm talking about, as there are very few of these children around anymore who demonstrate these character traits. Children of today don't even seem to know what they need, much less have the drive to go and get it. If it doesn't involve technology, they aren't interested. Children with internal motivation and drive – survive, and those who don't – perish. They perish in ways involving taking risks that lead to fatal accidents, getting depressed and suicidal, alcohol poisoning or drug overdoses, under-eating and dying of anorexia, or overeating and dying of obesity related factors. Lack of inner drive and motivation are but a few of the results of our technology driven culture, occurrences that are escalating and soon will be pandemic in the later 21st century.

The advent of technology has almost eliminated child inner drive or motivation to succeed - well, succeed at anything other than technology. The fast pace and immediate gratification that technology offers to children is eliminating their ability to wait for anything. As technology continually fuels the need for new and exciting experiences, patience for structured and routine tasks become a dying trait. I observe this universal impatience in children over and over in both homes and school settings as they "tantrum" their way toward behavior diagnoses and medication. Novelty is one of the many requirements for today's child, which is making teaching these children exceedingly difficult. As children require more and more fast paced and novel stimuli with which to capture their ever-diminishing attention spans, parents and teachers "ramp up" their use of technology. In a "last ditch" effort to educate these technology altered children, parents and teachers are choosing a methodology which may in the long term actually cause their demise. Building internal motivation and drive for non-technology related tasks and learning is difficult, but it can be done. Anything can be reversed, if we want to.

How to Foster Inner Drive

The term "inner drive" had its inception in sensory integration theory development by Dr. Jean Ayres in the late 1960's and early 1970's. Dr. Ayres was a researcher and occupational therapist who taught her student therapists how to "awaken" children through careful and meticulous adherence to what she termed a "just right challenge" concept. Dr. Ayres believed that a child exposed to tasks that were too easy, was under challenged and became resistant and bored, while a child who was given tasks they perceived to be too hard, suffered from anxiety and fright. Neither of these children could pay attention, as their energy states were either under or over aroused, thus prohibiting learning. Although she is now deceased, Dr. Ayres' concepts are still applied to children today, in order to build confidence in their skills and improve their desire to succeed. I often wonder what Dr. Ayres would think if she were to observe children today. Likely she would not have supported the use of technology by young children for the very reasons I am discussing now, the consequent destruction of desire for anything other than the technology itself.

In our technology obsessed children, building inner drive requires that parents and teachers address what types of tasks we are asking our children to do, and whether they actually have the skills to do them. Many children have no other leisure activity than to sit down in front of a television, video game or computer and be a passive recipient to a barrage of high speed, violent stimuli. This type of sensory input has hard wired children's brains to only register the fast, and ignore the slow stimuli. Unfortunately, parents and teachers are classified by children as "slow stimuli", and therefore simply cannot come close to competing for children's attention with high speed technology. So when asking a child to perform a non-technology related task, either at home or school, the parent and teacher must first address either speeding up the required task, or slowing down the child. Speeding up a task is exhausting for parents and teachers, and may be the reason why so many adults are describing "burn out" with parenting and teaching today's children, and why they default to technology. Slowing down the child can only be achieved with balancing activities children need for growth and success, with technology use.

Wild Colts Make the Best Horses

I regularly treat children who have been diagnosed with adhd and prescribed medication, but whose parents are seeking alternatives to drugging their child. These children are charged with energy, and require intense stimulation to their tactile, vestibular and proprioceptive sensory systems to enable them to calm their high energy states. I explain to parents that while the child has become sedentary through use of technology, their child's body requires intense and continuous movement in order to develop and learn. While we have stopped moving, our children have an innate mechanism to push themselves toward activities they need for development. We can no more tell a child to sit still, than we can tell them to stop breathing. In fact for the developing child, movement is as important as is breathing!

I also tell the parents that if their child was born 100 years ago, their biological bodies would be aptly suited to be the lead horse on a hunt spotting buffalo, or the lead fisherman for the tribe spotting fish in the streams. They would also be highly prized members of their community, as they could carry the heaviest buffalo or load of fish back to their camp. John Breeding, psychologist, educator, activist and author of *The Wildest Colts Make the Best Horses* reports that these children whom we are diagnosing and medicating are our "best and finest", they just haven't adapted to our sedentary ways of life. Their bodies crave movement stimulation, and their sensory systems are finely tuned to pick up the most subtle of stimuli. Plopped into a desk and told to sit still, these children quickly receive diagnoses for bad behavior, and stimulants to deaden their inner drive to excel.

Of course, the way to slow these adhd children down quick is to restrain them through the use of technology. These adhd children need to move, and respond best to lots of vestibular, proprioceptive, tactile and attachment stimulation. When adults start to manage a better balance between activities that promote child development and academic success with technology use, these children's bodies will be "primed" to access their minds. This concept is termed *Balanced Technology Management* and is discussed in its entirety in Section III of the *Virtual Child*. The way to manage this balance is through ensuring each individual child builds skill and confidence in a variety of activities, not just technology. Skill building involves not only exposure to varied activities, but also an exploration by each child into what sort of activities they value, prefer, and would like to pursue.

To help make this discovery process easier, I've developed a game called *Unplug'in* which helps children build skill and confidence in alternate activities to technology. *Unplug'in* is a board game that looks like a television, and the children are trapped inside and need to score points to get out. As the players travel through the *Me, We, Nature* and *Spirit* dimensions, they answer questions designed to learn more about themselves and their fellow players. Answering questions allows players to gather points necessary to travel to the *Victory Mile* to exit the game. Although *Unplug'in* can be played alone, the game was designed to be played with friends, family or classmates as a way to not only get to know more about themselves, but also about others, how they feel about nature, and what their relationship is with their spirit.

Reversing Learned Helplessness

All too often, in both home and school settings, children have the "task bar" set too high or too low; the former resulting in children who are bored and resistant, the later resulting in children who are anxious and afraid. Neither of these types of children can learn, and they quickly revert to what could be termed "helpless" behaviors: complaining, quitting a task without even trying, and never finishing a task. With 30% of children entering the school system developmentally delayed (Kershaw, 2009), the ability "gap" is widening to the point where it has become exceedingly difficult for the classroom teacher to accommodate the huge diversity of student abilities and variety of learning styles. Trying to get the "task bar" just right for 30 individual students is close to impossible. One of the most frequent reasons school systems use to justify the overuse of technology by struggling students is that they want to enable each individual to work at their own level and pace. While computers do offer students somewhat individualized programs, these programs are far from educational and are contributing to rising levels of illiteracy. So how do parents and educators offer tasks that have the ability bar and challenge set "just right"? In a nut shell, providing a range of tasks and individual choice is the way of the future in this new world of huge diversity of ability, but not through the use of computers. A range of tasks and individual choice won't work unless each child has found their inner drive to succeed. Section III will offer parents, educators and health professionals a variety of methods to address these problems.

There is one more missing link in building inner drive in our children. 21st century parents seem to have forgotten how to parent, and teachers how to teach. During individual discussions with both parents and teacher groups, I've discovered that many adults who work with children report they are actually *threatened* by technology, and truly believe that technology can entertain and educate their children better than they can. This erroneous belief, that parents and teachers are not "as good as" technology, is one of the largest contributing factors to our children loosing all sense of inner drive, and consequently adopting a "learned helpless" profile. Only when parents and teachers rediscover their own unique skills and abilities, and rebuild their confidence in parenting and teaching, will children discover the drive and motivation to participate in tasks. Even though the task might not be at their ability level, because they trust the skills and confidence of the task provider, they will attempt to do the work. Parents, grandparents, and teachers are *the most important people* in children's lives. If you don't think so, just ask your child! Resuming old salient roles and traditional family and education structures, will offer children the framework they need for achieving success at any task. Offering a variety of task levels and individual choice to accommodate different student skill levels, will be so much easier if these children have the necessary inner drive and motivation to initiate challenging tasks.

Inner Drive Directive
10 Steps to Ensure Self-Responsibility for Every Child

1. Create your *Inner Drive* Team

Commitment to establishing *Inner Drive* for all children will require that both parents and teachers come together to formulate a consistent and unified approach to achieving successful *Inner Drive* in children.

2. Reduce Technology Use

Infants and toddlers 0-2 years should NOT USE ANY forms of technology. Children age three and up, should not use more than two hours per day if the child appears to be developing "normally", and only one hour per day if child has developmental delays (American Academy of Pediatrics 2004).

3. Establish Movement Parameters

Children need to move: at least 3 hours per day for pre-school age children and 2-3 hours per day for elementary school age children. Increasing movement will not only promote optimal physical and mental development, but work to balance "energy in = energy out" necessary for optimal attention and learning. At home, children should balance every hour of technology use with an hour of physical activity, encouraging lots of heavy work and rough and tumble play. Wrestling or dance night family competitions are great ways to increase movement in fun and creative ways. Playground and community park equipment should enhance development and integration of children's balance, strength and touch sensory systems.

4. Seeing the Big Picture

The most salient motivator for human behavior is the perception that children are a productive part of the big picture. It is crucial for each child to have a sense that they will make an integral contribution to the world in their lifetime, and parents and teachers can teach them how! Often young children have no idea or concept of the individual contribution or special role they have within their family or classroom unit. Helping children find their own unique talents, will ensure they have a voice and something important to say. Use of art, music, song, dance and drama will give them a basis from which to flower, and for their imagination to flourish. Every child should feel that if they didn't exist, their family or classroom would fall apart. Give every child one job to do each day, and expect them to do it!

5. Just Right Challenge

The way children learn is by making mistakes. Children can reduce their fear of making mistakes through established daily periods of unstructured play that occurs without judgment or criticism. "Scribbling" is one example of a task that is unstructured and ungraded, and actually is a precursor to printing skill! When faced with a task that is perceived to be beyond a child's skill level, frustration and poor self-esteem will be the result. *Learned Helplessness* often plagues the grade three child, as children who repeatedly fail simply just *give up*. Each child should be able to find one thing they do really well, and then teach this skill to the rest of their family members and classmates.

6. Nurture Creativity

It's okay to make mistakes, this is how children establish and learn to value original ideas. Add activities into a child's life that don't require advanced skills or lots of practice. Music, art, dance, treadmills, exercise bikes, non-competitive games and silly skits in drama class can allow all children to participate without the bar being "too high" or "too low". Creativity is the basis of language content, and needs to be fostered. Once children's bodies establish rhythm and movement, the learning of other subjects in school is greatly enhanced. Don't leave our brightest kids behind!

7. Respect Individual Interest and Value Systems

Not all children are interested in or value the same activities as their parents and teachers think they should. While we want to foster tolerance for differences, respecting individual preferences can go a long way toward promoting motivation and *Inner Drive*. Design activities that allow children to individuate and identify their own unique interest and value systems. Offer variety and choice whenever possible, allow freedom of movement, and let go of conformity!

8. Balance Predictable Structure with Novelty

Predictable habits and routines allow the sensory system to relax and become less reactive. Novel situations foster adaptability. Predictability without novelty creates a very demanding, rigid child. Novelty without predictability creates a hyper-vigilant, reactive child. The job of parents and teachers is to skillfully *dance* the child between predictable structure and novelty.

9. Teach Zone'in Body Learning Concepts and Experience Zone'in Tools and Techniques

Use the *Zone'in Program*, including *Zone-O-Meters*, *Zone'in DVD*, *Zone'in Posters* and loads of *Zone'in Tools* and *Techniques* to teach children *Zone'in Concepts*, and then how to *Know* and then *Tone* their energy states. Establish *Zone'in Stations* with *Zone'in Tools* and *Techniques* in homes, classrooms and playgrounds. Then, get those kids *Zone'in to Learn!*

10. Expect Responsible Behavior!

Now that children understand their own unique contribution to the world, and have learned self regulation concepts from the *Zone'in Program*, parents should *expect* children to use responsible and self-regulatory techniques to ensure optimal energy states for attention and learning. Prior to starting homework or class work, parents and teachers should allow children two minutes to get their body energy *Zone'in to Learn*, and then back off and expect performance!

Nature

At the top of the list, "child safety" ranks as one of the paramount worries by parents all over the globe. Media reports of child deaths from abductions, accidents, sickness and murder travel on the internet like wild fire, striking fear in hearts and minds of everyone, parent or not. Watching what goes on around the world over and over on a variety of different networks and devices, ingrains horrific visual images forever in the memories of parents. The result of media's effective and efficient messaging to parents is a profound and griping *fear*, a fear that something horrible could happen to their own child. So parents keep their children indoors, clinging to them to keep them "safe" from whatever is out there.

We have become a fear-based society, a fact which rings true also in our schools and communities. Whether it's fear of child accidents, or fear of the resulting litigation, playgrounds have devolved into structures that only the toddlers find interesting. 21st century fear manufactured through multimedia, is *hyping* up parents to the extent that they are producing a whole generation of children who are literally immobilized by fright and anxiety. Unfortunately, these pervasive "fears" have distanced children from what could be the resolution to the dilemma of technology overuse, accessing the healing and restorative aspects of being outdoors in nature, and it is not just the fresh air that I'm talking about.

Richard Louv in his 2005 book *Last Child in the Woods – Saving Our Children From Nature-Deficit Disorder* reports that nature has an enormous capacity to calm the most anxious child, pacify anger and aggression, treat depression, reduce obesity, improve attention and learning, and optimize child development. The sensory aspects of nature, the smells, sounds, visual images, and tactile feelings are rarely experienced anymore, (watching nature shows doesn't count). When we drive past parks, or through residential neighborhoods, we no longer hear the joyous laughter or screams of delighted children. In fact, children are the universal missing factor in outdoor and nature environments today, but at what cost to their development and long term health?

This section of *Virtual Child* will explore the concept of child safety, and how the belief and fear that the world is "unsafe" is separating children from nature, causing irreparable damage to child health and well being. This section will also discuss the how the healing and attention restorative aspects of "green space" found in nature can reverse the detrimental aspects of technology on children.

Chapter 19

Child Safety and Nature – Are They Mutually Exclusive?

Burdette found in 2005 that parent's perception of safety positively correlates with the amount of technology their child uses. What this means is that if a parent perceives the world as "unsafe", their child is likely to become exposed to significantly more television, video games and internet use than a parent who generally thinks the world is "safe". A very important task for parents and teachers everywhere, is to discuss with each other, and then discuss with their children, individual perceptions regarding safety. Only then will families and schools be able to make reasonable (not impassioned) decisions regarding what is safe and what is not safe. For example, is it safe for a 10 year old to ride their bike to the school or park? All too often we make *absolute* rules, often when children are young, and then never question these rules as the child gets older. Strict adherence to a rule made when a child was 5 years of age, likely has no validity when the child turned 10, but it is still "the rule". Keeping children safe isn't about keeping them inside, it's about maximizing safety and minimizing risk, but not at the expense of limiting or restricting exposure to activity that children need to optimize growth and success.

A question to ask of children in both home and classroom-based settings is "What do you think is safe?" and "What are you afraid of?" This information will help parents and teachers to determine if their child's fears are realistic, or have their fears been "adopted" from what they have read in media, heard about at home, or talked about with peers on the playground. Some of the areas a family or classroom discussion should cover could follow the *"who, what, when where, why* and *how"* scenario. For example, should an eight year old child be able to ride their bike to their friend's house? If not, at what age might this activity be deemed "safe" by both child and parents? Would there be a way to make this activity safe, for example riding their bike with an older sibling or a friend? Should a four year old play outside alone in a fenced backyard? If this thought turns parent's stomachs into a swarm of butterflies, then how might they be able to modify this activity to ensure all concerns are met?

By sitting down with family members, school-based teams and classrooms, and addressing everyone's perception of fear, these tough and scary thoughts are not so scary after all. I'm certainly not telling readers what type of restrictions to place on their children to ensure their safety, but I am suggesting that readers challenge their present belief system regarding safety, and possibly question some of the existing rules to determine whether they are valid and reasonable. Again, we want to minimize risk and maximize safety, but not to the detriment of development.

Everyone knows, but few remember the fact that statistically, it is family members and close friends who abduct and murder children, not strangers. Therefore, one of the best assurances parents can have of child safety is to be aware of who they are spending their time with. How well do you know your new friend you just met? Trust your instincts, and don't let suspicious or dangerous people come into your or your child's life. While this may seem to be quite simple and logical information, it's surprising how many parents don't listen when the internal alarm bells go off in their minds about someone. A simple call to the police or child services to check someone out that you are suspicious about, might go a long way towards keeping your child safe and out of harm's way.

Fear of Nature

It has been a long time since I have seen a "dirty" child. I remember treating children 15 years ago who looked as if they had stepped right out of a mud puddle. Today's children are not only "clean" in the morning, but they somehow manage to stay that way all day! My bothers, neighborhood friends, and I used to go outside in the morning and come back home at night *filthy*. I grew up next to Puget Sound in Washington, and our "playground" in the summer was the beach. We spent so much time in the salt chuck that our ankles were literally *green* in color most of the summer from the seaweed. We were healthy, happy and so tired at night that we would collapse in bed and sleep like babies. Many of today's well meaning parents erroneously think that germs live in the dirt. They don't. Germs live on people, and exposing children to the outside world of nature will serve to *protect*, not *harm* children. This realization that "outdoors is good" has now permeated many of the Canadian and United States day care and preschool communities who have created licensing standards for daily outside play.

Back in the early 1970's, there was tremendous movement in North America to claim forest land for the creation of community, state and provincial parks. While the majority of these parks exist to this day, park attendance is at an all time low. Cub Scout participation in both Canada and the United States is half of what it was 20 years ago. Why is this? People just don't value nature anymore, or at least not as much as they value the allure of their various devices. Viewing nature shows or pictures on the internet seems to fulfill the call of nature in today's world.

In his book *Last Child in the Woods*, Richard Louv draws links between the absence of nature in the lives of today's "wired generation" to the rise in obesity, attention disorders and depression. Louv describes how many adults and their children, now view nature as the "Bogeyman", a place to be feared, which he describes is a belief far from any truth. Movies like *The Blair Witch Project* where bad and very scary things happen to a group of hikers, has done great damage through imbedding viewers memories with visual images they will re-experience over and over. As I am an avid kayak camper and scuba diver, I will never see *The Blair Witch Project*, nor have I ever seen *Jaws* as I know scary memories would follow me into the woods and the sea. I am constantly warning parents that their child's mind is like a camera and will remember forever what they watch – especially *The News!* Can you imagine what a young infant or toddler might think when viewing people being blown apart by bombs, or looking at dead and lifeless bodies? They are horrified, and quite likely these images are what they are seeing when they can't go to sleep at night or wake with nightmares. Children carry these images wherever they go, yet somehow parents think that their children are safer "inside".

Healing Aspects of Nature

My experiences with nature go way back to my early childhood and continue to this day. If I skip my twice daily walk with my two dogs Jack and Henry, I am grouchy and have great difficulty concentrating on anything other than mundane tasks. My "nature breaks" are times when I am able to "download" all the information I've been processing all day, and are major contributors to why I can so easily go to sleep, and stay asleep all night. I feel more "safe" walking through the forests surrounding my house than I do crossing a parking lot in Vancouver! I've faced bears, cougars, coyotes and wolves many times and without incident. A night time walk in nature is not near as scary for me as walking around at night in large cities. I've been able to share my love of nature many times over with my children, in many unique and wonderful ways.

When my daughter was two years old, she "saw" two fairies in the forest near our house; one with white skin wearing a pink dress, and one with brown skin wearing a white dress. Since that time we and others have built over 14 structures for her fairies, bringing in friends and classmates over the years to complete the village. Children from as far as the interior of British Columbia knew about the *Sandy Hook Fairy Village*, and would bring special gifts and leave them for the fairies whenever they came to the Sunshine Coast. Unfortunately someone did not like our fairy forest glen, and the whole village disappeared overnight. Every building was flattened and hidden behind a downed tree, and every gift for the fairies taken away and apparently destroyed. This was a tragedy of epic proportion for my daughter, who was interviewed by the local paper about what she thought might have happened. She was a wee five year old at the time, and reported she had nightmares about her fairies lying about bleeding, with their wings torn off, dying. My daughter and her friends, as well as all the Moms and Dads who helped build the *Fairy Village*, were quite upset and have never forgotten this tragedy. But fairies are indomitable and do live on, and a new fairy village has reappeared in a safer and more secluded glen, and new structures continue to be built to this day.

Nature is and has always been a special friend in my life and the lives of my children. The new age way of moving our children away from nature will leave our children alone and sad. Parents helping children to understand and experience nature and her tremendous beauty and ability to calm the most anxious child, will help their children to discover a magical and wonderful experience like no other.

Attention Restoration and Nature

Dr. S. Kaplan is a well known researcher on the subject of "attention restoration". He discovered in 1995 that whenever a child's attention is "taxed", there needs to be a period of time where the child is allowed to "restore" their attention. Kaplan proposed that balancing attention *taxing* activities with attention *restoration* activities is essential to optimize attention and learning states. Kaplan's theories blend nicely with work by Anne Fabor-Taylor who in 2004 discovered that inner city children have three times the adhd as rural children. In an excellent research study design, Dr. Faber-Taylor and her research partner Dr. Kuo found in 2007 that it was the amount of "green space" that a child is exposed to that determines the extent their attention is restored. In school settings, green space can be accessed by a child simply opening a window and taking a long deep breath of fresh air, while looking at the trees, grass or shrubs. Living in remote Northern locations, where environments are either brown or white, is a challenge to accessing green space. Bringing plants into classrooms, or growing a garden in a greenhouse solarium or conservatory attached to the school, would improve children's attention and learning by exposing them to the attention restorative aspects of nature. Children could visit these "green" areas when they need to calm or recharge their energy bodies.

Schools planning student daily access of 20 minutes per day to "green space", would effectively counteract the "overload" effects of technology use, promoting focused attention and learning. Green space is defined as nature-based and alive, including plants, shrub, trees, grass, and flowers, and can be created either indoors, or accessed outdoors.

Indoor green space is already accessible to classrooms with a view of nature, which a number of studies have now shown it can produce students with lower behavior problems and higher academic performance. Fresh air breaks, either through opening the window or door to the outside, can prove to be essential techniques for students who are lethargic in the afternoon. Indoor green space can also be designed and achieved through use of greenhouse-type environments such as arboretums, conservatories and biospheres that contain aspects of nature e.g. plants, small trees, ponds with waterfall, patch of grass. Funds might be accessed for creation of indoor green space through local community groups and organizations, or alternatively, through application to technology production corporations.

Outdoor green space can be accessed during recess and lunch breaks with strict adherence given to the policy of no technology use during these designated time periods. Accessing outdoor space for a short time prior to tests or more difficult subjects such as math, can prove to be an effective strategy to ensure optimal learning. Starting a school gardening project with daily access to shoveling a bit of dirt would not only provide green space access, but also provide necessary proprioceptive input for calming an aggressive or anxious child. Weekly field trips to a local park, woods, farm or beach, and/or yearly classroom or school camping trips would provide children with a more significant experience of the soothing aspects of nature. Accessing *Mother Nature* feeds not only the body and mind, but also the soul, and is truly the best remedy for problems associated with technology overuse.

In moving our children toward sustainable futures, and creating healthy environments that support attention and learning, it is imperative that schools embrace increased access to nature, as well as movement, touch and human connection strategies. Children who "act out" are simply *craving* movement, touch and human connection, and the only way they know how to get their needs met is be *extreme* in their behavior. Otherwise, who would listen to them? All behavior has meaning, and it is our job as parents, teachers and therapists to determine what a child is try to say with their "behavior". Plugging these children into technology, or diagnosing and medicating them, might be a "quick fix", but it is also an intervention that is likely to "back fire" in a very short time.

Reaching out with a kind word and deep pressure touch techniques, or encouraging a child to run on a treadmill or play with a wobble board, can not only calm an anxious child, but also enable that child to pay attention and learn. Employing attention restorative strategies of access to nature and movement is one essential step that will successfully take schools into the new millennium, creating sustainable futures for all children.

Chapter 20

Recess and Playgrounds - The Epicenter for Child Development and Learning

In the best of homes, schools and communities, accidents do happen. But employing a "knee jerk" response of dramatically lowering the height of slides and swings, and taking merry-go-rounds (remember those?) to the dump is neither wise nor called for to ensure child safety. Alternatively, there are a number of steps parents, education and health professionals can take to prevent and reduce the number of accidental fatalities and injuries. Minimizing risk and maximizing safety are tenants we should strive for in the design of safe spaces for children to play. The *Canadian Standards Association* sets rules for playgrounds, and if followed can halve the playground injury rate (MacAurthur, 2000). Environmental modifications, such as creation of adequate fall space and fall surface, can reduce injury rates by 50-75% (Howard, 2010). So we don't need to turn our playgrounds into structures that would challenge only the toddler generation, we can through careful design create interesting and fun play areas for all ages.

The Importance of Recess

While recess is an essential part of a child's day for socialization and physical activity, many children are allowed technology use during recess, gravely limiting opportunity for movement, touch and human connection. Another limitation to movement on the playground is the fact that one in three children are obese, and one in three children are developmentally delayed. These children don't readily join in playground socializing and movement activities at recess, as these activities are difficult and often embarrassing to perform. Children who are obese or delayed in their development require activities that offer challenge, but that are not so taxing to their physical systems that it discourages them from participating. Offering access to treadmills, exercise bikes or stair climbers during recess and lunch periods, would provide children with physical limitations an opportunity to challenge themselves to beat their personal "best". This equipment would best be located outside to optimize attention restoration, sheltered from wind and rain under a porch covered area such as a overhang or extended roof.

Recess durations are another issue of concern in today's schools. In a study which looked at 11,000 third-graders ages 8-9 years, Dr. R M Barros found that those children who had greater than 15 minutes per day of recess, had teacher reports of better classroom behavior. Dr. Barros's study also found that over 30% of students had little or no recess (< 15 minutes per day), and 40% of the schools surveyed reportedly had cut back at least one daily recess period. Since the 1970's, children have lost 12 hours per week in free time, with grave effects on their developmental level, and consequently their ability to perform academically. With all that we know now about the positive effects of movement on a child's ability to learn, twice daily recess, in addition to a break at lunch time, should be mandatory in all schools. Cutting back on recess and increasing academic loads is a proven recipe for failure, both academically and behaviorally. Well functioning classrooms are those with frequent breaks (both in and outdoors) and organized recess activities with a variety of equipment to challenge children who might have obesity or developmental delays. These types of activities are supported in the classroom with self regulation programs such as the *Zone'in Program* to enhance motivation, attention and learning.

Minimal Standards for Playground Structures

With one third of a child's day spent sedentary, homes, schools and communities can provide organized activity on playground structures that provide critical sensory and motor challenges to improve child development and academic performance. Playground structures have changed markedly over the past decade, largely due to litigation concerns by schools and communities. Slides and swings are shorter, merry-go-rounds non-existent, and trapeze bars, jungle gyms and overhead parallel bars are a fading memory. Gyms have lost their climbing ropes, ladders, uneven parallel bars, springs and horses. These changes to child play and physical education structures have come at a detriment to child development. Children are not receiving the type of sensory and motor input they need for adequate neurological development and academic performance, impacting further on their ability to print, read and pay attention. Safety can be achieved, while still significantly challenging a child's sensory and motor system.

Playground structures should contain elements that contribute to the development of the sensory and motor systems. This equipment can be placed inside homes, back yards, gyms, under outdoor covered areas, or on school and community playgrounds. Every play station or playground should have at least four devices that stimulate *each* of the following three sensory systems, located either indoors or outdoors, and accessed by *every* student on a daily basis:

Vestibular System – *Posture and Arousal*

Equipment that causes a child to move off their centre of gravity serves to activate the vestibular system, which in turn activates core stabilizer muscles, bringing the child back into their center and facilitating midline postural tone. This strong core is required for integration of both sides of the body, and coordination of both eyes. Vestibular stimulation also optimizes a child's arousal state, enabling attention. Examples of playground vestibular equipment would be a variety of types of swings (frog, traditional, hammock, platform, tire, inner tube, rope, disc), trapeze bars, zip lines, slides, merry-go-rounds, trampolines, spring rockers, gliders, therapy balls, spin boards (can make with two pieces of plywood and Lazy Susan), plastic spin discs, and scooter boards.

Proprioceptive System – *Strength and Coordination*

Equipment that makes a child's muscle and joint systems work hard activates the proprioceptive system, which promotes strength and coordination of the muscles, and also serves to calm down a child who is agitated and aggressive. Examples of playground proprioceptive equipment would be a variety of types of climbing devices (ropes, cargo net, frames, climbing mounts on walls), jungle gyms, parallel bars, pulling on deflated bicycle inner tubes (get from local bike shop), Tug-Of-War rope (children who fight should be required to do a Tug-Off), crawling through plastic tubes, chin-up bars, and exercise bikes.

Tactile System – *Praxis and Calming*

Equipment that administers deep pressure touch to the mechanoreceptors found in a child's tactile or touch system, serves to help that child know where their body is in space, a precursor for planning specific movement patterns essential for fine and gross motor tasks known as "praxis". Examples of playground tactile equipment would be lycra pod swings, crawling inside large inflated truck tire inner tubes, rolling children tight in blankets (called "burrito"), rolling down grassy slopes, crawling through lycra tubes, getting squished in between two bean bag chairs or gym mats, and running and jumping onto a large duvet cover filled with foam chips (get from local foam shop).

Litigation and Safety

If playgrounds are in disrepair or substandard, parents are advised to meet with school administrations and community centers regarding designing of playgrounds that would ensure safety, while promoting necessary movement. While safety is an important consideration, rough and tumble play will result in occasional injuries to children, as evidenced by the children lining up for ice bags at the school office during recess. Minimizing these injuries requires not only careful planning and design of playground structures, but also planning around traffic flow patterns, and frequent playground equipment training sessions with students. A few considerations might be ensuring the following:

- adequate fall space – the higher they climb, the wider arc they fall
- absorbent surface – pea gravel, rubber matting, bark, grass
- all season safety – sun (hot), rain (wet), snow (removal, visual occlusion), sleet (slippery)
- vandalism – may need to do nightly removal

While maximizing safety and minimizing injuries are important, these two goals should not be achieved at the risk of jeopardizing child development. Three great websites for information regarding creating safe playgrounds are *Safe Kids Canada, United States Consumer Product Safety Commission*, and the *Canadian Standards Associations*.

The *Zone'in* website zonein.ca has a one hour webinar titled "Safe Playground Design" to assist parents, schools and communities in building playgrounds that challenge a child's sensory and motor development, while also minimizing risk for injury and maximizing safety. We can do this.

Chapter 21

Choosing the Path of People and Nature

Words of Wisdom from a Native Elder

Traditional people of Indian nations have interpreted the two roads that face the light-skinned race as the road to technology and the road to spirituality. We feel that the road to technology.... has led modern society to a damaged and seared earth.

Could it be that the road to technology represents a rush to destruction, and that the road to spirituality represents the slower path that the traditional native people have traveled and are now seeking again?

The earth is not scorched on this trail. The grass is still growing there.

William Commanda, Mamiwinini, Canada, (1991)

Zone'in and First Nations Schools

During the past twenty years as a pediatric occupational therapist, I've had the opportunity to work in many diverse environments with hundreds of children, but I've never truly experienced the wonderful spirit of First Nation's children until May of 2009. In a small village in northern British Columbia, where transportation is by snowmobile and field trips are ice fishing and 40 kilometers "bush whacking" treks, lives a school full of warm hearted children who despite numerous obstacles, were absolutely a delight to work with. Living close to the land seemed to enable these children to more easily access their inner drive and sense of spirit needed to succeed and perform. These children made my heart soar each and every day.

Many of these children initially appeared quite shy and withdrawn. Use of a variety of vestibular, proprioceptive, tactile, and attachment tools and techniques, quickly brought these children's spirit and joy back into their hearts and eyes. The impact of my work to enable these children to access their innate ability and accept the challenge to perform academically, was nothing short of wonderful. Calm and centered, many of the children were finally able to *output* mountains of "buried" knowledge. The ability to "ground" their energy and "prime" their bodies for learning finally allowed these brilliant children access to the power of their mind.

Special Education Teacher Dialogue

After attending Cris's workshop on the Zone'in Program, myself and another teacher, started to look at the different ways we could bring the program into our classrooms. My colleague had the most structured approach. She showed the video to her students about once a week. The students loved the movie. Their favorite scene in the movie was when the characters dressed up and completed the chores that children would have had to do 100 years ago. In this skit stuffed animals were roasted over a fake fire and that always got a laugh.

While watching the movie weekly, my colleague put a pencil box in each child's desk with things they could chew or fiddle with. She also set up a corner in her room where the children were allowed to get in the Zone during particular times of the day. She found that many of her students used and academically benefited from the new tools.

I found it was very obvious that certain students needed certain tools. Two of my boys went for chewies, while another girl immediately wanted earplugs. Overall the experience opened up a new relationship between teacher and student as us teachers were continuously trying to see if adjusting sensory stimulation could help our students focus. And the students started to understand self-regulation. It was a start.

After working on our own with the Zone'in Program, we invited Cris up to our school in May because we wanted her to help us work with our more extreme kids. Cris did a great job. She gave us a lot of practical exercises which we were able to implement right away. We tied rubber tubing to some of the desks so the students could pull really hard while they had their feet up against their desk legs. One boy who was so angry at life that he often shut down, was able to put his anger into pulling on this band while doing his math. For another boy just doing the hand push from the video on his own was not enough and he has learned to come up daily and ask me to stick my hands out so he could push on them. This same boy also frequently requests that a lot of weight be placed on his shoulders. These activities have helped these boys be more calm and attentive in their classrooms. There are so many other examples I will just briefly list a few more:

1. *A student diagnosed with FAS hated doing his school work. He would roll his head on his desk stating "It hurts". Cris helped me to see that he was seeking "pressure" on his forehead to enable him to focus. After allowing him this pressure, and giving him other types of pressure devices and techniques, this student was able to concentrate on his reading and was motivated to do so.*

2. *An student diagnosed with ADD frequently "climbed the walls" and hung from door frames in school. This was very distracting to other children in the classroom. Cris suggested we use 22kg weights as an energy outlet and to "ground" his energy, which calmed his body and enabled him to settle down and do his work. This student stated he didn't like being in the Zone because he was not used to it. Because of his living situation, he needs to be out of his body, but the weights do work when he uses them.*

The above discoveries have all come from the Zone'in Program and Cris's visit to our school.

The Zone'in Program opens up dialogue for self-regulation between teacher and student, which is a good starting point. For some of our students, the program alone did increase their academic output, but most of the students I work with as a Special Education Teacher are way more "out of the Zone" than the students in the video. I think First Nations Steering Association (FNSA) Schools and their students would benefit from having Cris revamp her Zone'in video for First Nations Schools.

My overall suggestions for a First Nations Zone'in Video:

Have First Nations Children in the video and the more footage we can get of remote village schools the better it will connect with those kids.

Perhaps more consideration to the activity level of the First Nations Children who live in remote villages (many of them do live in the bush at times during the year, so I wonder how many hours of T.V these children watch)?

Show older and younger students in a classroom setting.

Watching Cris with my students was when I learned the most, and after a few sessions I started to see patterns on my own. The new video could have a section on some common symptoms that our students exhibit when they are out of the Zone and some ideas on how to get them back in. This section should also include some of the more extreme behavior and how we can use the Zone'in concepts.

I realize that getting in the Zone is not prescriptive, but I think that by watching how other students energy levels can get out of control, and then watching another adult work with that student, would help many of us educators.

Working with Cris has been amazing. She is knowledgeable, flexible and passionate about her work and I think FNSA schools could benefit from having her tailor Zone'in for First Nations Students.

Jessica McKerrow, Special Education Teacher, British Columbia

SECTION III

Solutions - Creating Sustainable Futures with Balanced Technology Management

Sustainability Through Balance

You must be the change you want to see in the world.

Mahatma Gandhi

Section I and II of the *Virtual Child* documented an incremental rise in personal use of entertainment technology, with the consequence of not meeting critical milestones for child sensory and motor development and/or attainment of literacy. I discussed how parental time spent connected to technology is disconnecting parents from their children, causing a rise in attachment and behavior disorders. As traditional family systems and structures disintegrate, isolated and lonely children consequently form unhealthy attachments with technology. Educators in the school system are escalating their use of computers as tools for teaching children without evidence to support this initiative, nor sufficient research regarding long term outcomes. As limited education funding is diverted to technology, playgrounds – the epicenter for socialization and child development - fall into disrepair.

In Section III of *Virtual Child*, readers will be guided toward an approach that practices *managing balance* between activities children need to grow and succeed with their use of technology. Development of *Balanced Technology Management Foundation Teams* from six different sectors, and enactment of specific initiatives by each sector, will ensure sustainable futures for the children of the 21st century. Bringing together representatives from six target sectors: parent, teacher, health professional, government, research, and technology production corporations, will provide communities with a wide range of ideas and plans for achieving management between activities children need to grow and succeed, with technology use. Whether operating on a large or small scale, *Foundation Teams* will be the first step toward reversing the trend of children overusing technology. If we do nothing, nothing will change. If we start by forming teams of like-minded individuals to begin planning, change is just around the corner.

No matter what peril befalls the human race, the term "balance" could be applied as an effective and often efficient solution. Extreme measures and initiatives rarely work, as the energy required to implement them over long periods of time is just too great. Minimalist measures are generally just "not enough". It is only when human beings achieve *balance* between two opposing forces that evolution proceeds. Section III will profile solutions required to address the problem of technology overuse by children, and present a variety of methods and theories that can be applied in home, school and community settings. This section contains useful tools and techniques that parents, teachers, health professionals, government, researchers, and technology production corporations can utilize to manage and balance technology use and create sustainable futures for all children.

Who Will Be the Foundation Team Players?

Relying on parents to impose technology restrictions on their children may not prove to be an effective strategy in all situations, as child technology usage patterns often parallel that of their parents (Jordan, 2006). Furthermore, evidence suggests some parents may have technology addictions themselves (Horvath, 2004). These conditions support inclusion of a variety of professionals from different sectors who either work with, or on behalf of children, in order to manage balance between activities children need to grow and succeed, with their use of technology. The health and education systems could work together to screen children for technology overuse, and provide information for families on effective technology management methods. The routine use of the *Technology Screen* by primary care physicians, pediatricians, psychologists, psychiatrists, social workers, occupational and physical therapists, speech and language pathologists, and even those who work in the education sector is imperative to identify children who overuse technology. As only a small segment of the population accesses the health care system on a regular basis, the education system is likely the best avenue for distribution of technology management information. Brochures or handouts could be sent home with children, or education could be provided to parents during school meetings or parent education sessions

I suggest that governments and researchers work together to develop technology usage guidelines, and then pass this crucial information onto parents, health and education professionals. Because of the rapid speed of technology development we will always be delayed in receiving the most current research information needed to guide policy decisions. There is adequate research at this time for government to move forward and mandate risk warnings on technology products, and create guidelines for safe usage of technology in home and school-based settings. Government and researchers need to work more closely to regulate technology production corporations regarding product safety for children. While it is ultimately up to the parent to determine the type and usage parameters of technology for their child, providing parents with more information on the inherent risks of using these products is essential and currently lacking. This area of "informed risk" is ripe for potential litigation, as parents have a right to receive up to date information from not only technology production corporations, but also from researchers and government regarding product safety and risk.

Chapter 22

Creating Sustainable Futures Programs

Your future is created by what you do today, not tomorrow.

Robert Kiyosaki

While readers may be thinking I am against all use of technology, I'm not. Technology is, for better or worse, the way of the future for our children. Parents and teachers just need to learn how to prioritize engagement in activities children need to grow and succeed, and prioritize these activities over technology use. While some adults might find this task daunting, achieving critical factors for child development and academic success is actually quite easy, with a plan. Key players who work with children will be invited to come together as a team to plan, implement and eventually manage this "balance" between child activity and technology. Section III contains such a plan, the *Creating Sustainable Futures Program*, which has two key components:

1. **Creation of *Foundation Teams***

The first stage in the *Creating Sustainable Futures Program* is the formation of local community *Balanced Technology Management Foundation Teams* composed of key players from six different target sectors. I've listed examples of possible team members from each of the six target sectors below. This list is obviously endless, and consists of primary members who might be interested in the area of creating sustainable futures for children. This list is not complete by any means, but is a place to start for future planning of managing balanced technology use.

- **Parents** – parent advisory councils, support groups, foster parents organizations, or retired grandparent groups.
- **Educators** – school boards, school technology managers, special education coordinators, principals, early child education managers.
- **Health Professionals** – professional associations, local health units, children's hospitals and rehabilitation centers, child care centers, licensing boards.
- **Government** – policy makers from health, education and children and family ministries and government branches.
- **Researchers** – early education, child development, pharmaceutical, child health, child education, attachment.
- **Technology Production Corporations** – video game designers, public relations, research, legal departments, education.

As *Foundation Teams* become more prolific, a movement of epic proportion will begin to take shape, and our voices will grow to immeasurable heights.

2. **Identification of *Balanced Technology Management* Initiatives**

While each Foundation Team can create their own *Balanced Technology Management* initiatives that would be specific to the population served, generalized and universal concepts for each of these six sectors are to follow. These general initiatives can serve as a template to assist the *Foundations Teams* in their initial stages of planning and design for specific population based initiatives for each of the six sectors.

Enactment of *Balanced Technology Management* initiatives would be most effective with inclusion of highly skilled professionals, such as occupational therapists to provide community based workshops and programs. I have developed six *Foundation Series Workshops* for parents, educators and health professionals, as well as have designed a variety of programs to assist in enactment of *Balanced Technology Management* initiatives. I've also developed an instructor training module for occupational therapists who would like to teach the *Foundation Series Workshops*.

Through the formation of the *Balanced Technology Management Foundation Teams*, and development and enactment of specific initiatives within each target sector, the "technology train" can be slowed down and brought back to the station. This will provide much needed time to assess the immediate impact caused to children by technology overuse, and determine immediate and long term planning and interventions. Taking time now, to accurately assess the damage technology has already caused our children, will enable us to better plan for responsible technology use in the future.

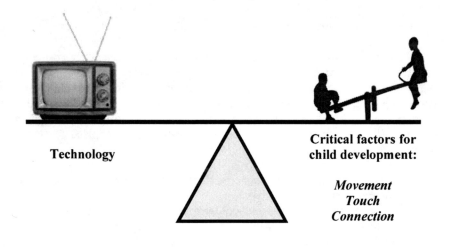

Technology

Critical factors for child development:

Movement
Touch
Connection

Chapter 23

Reducing the Use vs. Managing Balance

We cannot become what we need to be by remaining what we are.

Max Depree

When I first became concerned about the results of technology overuse by children, I spoke in terms of "reducing the use", as opposed to "managing balance". The former concept was met with resistance, offence and down right anger, while the latter was more easily processed. When talking with any of my potential target *Foundation Team* members, whether they be from the parent, teacher, health professional, government, research or technology production corporation groups, everyone had a easier time accepting the term "balanced management" than discussing how they were going to get children to "reduce the use". I will expand on this concept of acceptance for the term "managing balance", with examples of experiences I have had with our six target sector groups. Readers will likely find this information useful when considering how they will proceed in addressing balanced technology use.

Parents – The Scapegoat or the Key to Success?

Everyone seemed to blame the parents when it came to problems associated with technology overuse. While parents are the ones who will set limits and restrictions, presently they are unaware of the extent of the problem. That said, I have provided over 200 workshops to education and health professionals, and always request the workshop organizer invite parents, but few actually attend unless the workshop is designated specifically for parents. Does this possibly mean that parents don't want to find out information that they are ill equipped to do anything about? Then we need to also provide parents with technology management tools and support. Changing whole family structures to accommodate restrictive rules regarding technology overuse may in some cases require extensive professional support. Technology – while designed to make life more efficient and entertaining, has resulted in stressed and busy lifestyles for today's families. What we need at this point in time is a trend setting "shift" in how we as a society, view technology. A "movement" of epic proportions is now required, and parents already are the leaders in this change.

When I speak to parents about technology overuse, I always preface this information by stating that technology is not a bad thing, it just has to be balanced with activity. Generally speaking, this approach has been met with a positive response. I am a believer in the power of the parent when provided with correct and useful information. I am also a believer in the power of children to make correct decisions for themselves when they have the facts and the tools to do so. If we teach parents how to ensure children engage in activities required for growth and success, then maybe children would acquire enough skills so they would want to "unplug" themselves. Parents, and their children, are the keys to the success of balanced management of technology, and likely will be the first members to form local *Balanced Technology Management Foundation Teams*.

Educators – Look Before You Leap

Educators are seriously immersed in the virtual realm, and are deeply under the "technology illusion" that a computer is an effective teaching tool for just about everyone. I have spoken to many educators who actively dispute my concern, especially the district technology managers whose job it is to push technology, and it seems like "more is better" as far as they are concerned. They do not appear to recognize the need for technology reduction, nor support balanced management. Technologies used today in school settings are lacking in evidence and long term outcomes. Even if a teacher does question whether technology is actually teaching anything to children, they are bound by the decisions of their administrators, school boards, and education governments who often are recommending more technology. Reducing the use of technology will be a hard sell to the school systems, and requires careful and accurate presentation of facts in order to help educators realize the damage technology use is inflicting on children. This is why I suggest including the school technology managers on the *Balanced Technology Management Foundation Teams*. Providing these essential team members with accurate information, will enable them to participate in development of realistic management initiatives.

Health Professionals – One Nation Under Therapy

While health professionals are definitely worried about children, they have also unknowingly created a diagnostic and medication "machine" that will be hard to turn around. Realizing that technology overuse is in some cases being diagnosed as a mental illness and medicated, is a first step. I received initial feedback from professional associations to whom I had submitted conference abstracts and journal articles, that my recommendations of adherence to expert guidelines was "unrealistic" e.g. dropping children down from 7.5 hours per day technology use to 1-2 hours per day. This reaction seemed strange, as they were not willing to support their colleague's recommendations. I hope that professional associations do not back off their original recommendations due to high technology usage, but rather look at how to create "baby steps" toward technology reduction, especially with our high users. I continue to be surprised at the general "dismissing" of the parent by the health professional in the realm of elevating themselves to a status of empirical knowledge. We are not the experts of a parent's child, and their child is not sick. By stopping the diagnostic and medication crisis, and instead offering parents education and support to manage technology use, the health professional can carve out a new advisory role for themselves as a parent advocate and builder of healthy attachments between parent and child.

Government – For Corporate Business, or *For the People*

Health and education governments are responsible for allowing technology to escalate unrestricted, and for not informing parents of the detrimental effects of technology. For the past three years I have been sending information to Education, Health and Children and Family Ministries in Canada regarding the impact of technology overuse by children. While I have received responses from many of these Ministers, the majority of their letters tell me about their new initiatives to make children more active at home and in schools, or talk about their new "wellness" campaigns. No one appeared to be interested in technology awareness programs, and not one Minister agreed to meet with me to discuss my concerns as requested. Conversations with Health Canada indicated that while they saw it as their mandate to be concerned in areas associated with electromagnetic radiation, some of the more pronounced effects of technology such as developmental delay and obesity, were not of interest to the department with which I was speaking.

In May of 2010 I was invited by our British Columbia Minister for Children and

Families, to present my concerns regarding technology's impact on the developing child, to policy development representatives from the Health, Education and Children and Family Ministries, which I did on May 21, 2010 in Victoria, BC. I hope to continue this practice of meeting with government representatives to offer information regarding a variety of initiatives in the health, education and children and family sectors. As a result of feedback obtained through the conference organizer, I created a one hour webinar for government representatives, currently available on the *Zone'in* website zonein.ca.

Researchers – Get to the Point

Over the past five years I have reviewed literally hundreds of research articles and government documents, and am stunned at the fact that rarely does child developmental research take into account technology overuse as a variable in research design. This seems striking, as technology has profound direct and indirect effects on child development and academic performance. About two years ago I created a database of child development researchers, and routinely now write to them advocating that they include child technology use as a research parameter. I have included in my requests that researchers consider a *Technology Screen* and use of the *Technology Guidelines* components, detailed in Section I of *Virtual Child*. While I did hear back from a few professors, predominantly stating it was an "interesting" request, many of them never responded. This failure to include the parameter of technology use in child research fails to "get to the point" considering many conditions under extensive study. Even if it's a study on asthma, why not ask how much technology the child is using? Who knows, maybe there is a link. If there has been research proven causality to technology already, for example regarding a condition such as obesity, it is unconscionable to not include *technology use* as a parameter in all obesity research. It is imperative to have representatives from the child researcher community on the *Balanced Technology Management Foundation Teams*.

Technology Production Corporations

Technology production corporations reported in conversations regarding overuse of technology by children, that they thought it was the responsibility of the parents to restrict technology use. If the parents indeed restricted use, then the technology product would likely not pose harm to their child. When I countered this argument that uniformed parents can't impose restrictions, as they don't have accurate information to raise the "alarm bells", the corporations reported they did not believe product risk information was their mandate. This poses problems, and likely requires government intervention. We had discussed concepts such as providing a webinar for their video game designers regarding critical factors for child development, in order that these factors could be taken into consideration with gaming design to reduce detrimental impact on children. As the number of "kills" in video games directly correlate with the level of consequent child aggression (Anderson, 2008), we discussed possible ways to limit the number of "kills". This could easily be achieved through changing different parameters of the game. For example sniper characters fire their weapons less frequently, complicated gun scope set-up, or diversion activities such as having to "bury their dead", could slow down the killing process. Partnerships between child development specialists and technology production corporations would be integral for ensuring children are not harmed in the process of using technology. Knowledgeable technology production corporations, working in conjunction with child development experts, could possibly even design technology that enhances, as opposed to negates, child physical, mental, social and academic performance.

Summary

Conversations with representatives from six target sectors, was integral in the formation of my recommended *Foundation Team* members, and *Balanced Technology Management* initiatives. These conversations to a large degree, determined why I've selected these specific six target groups as focal points for enacting initiatives. Key representatives working together to form these *Foundation Teams,* and adopting initiatives discussed in future chapters of *Virtual Child*, will successfully work toward reversing the detrimental effects of technology, and strive to create sustainable futures for all children. In the next chapter, I would like to accurately define *Balanced Technology Management*, and discuss how it would work in different environments to enhance child development and academic performance.

Chapter 24

Balanced Technology Management Concepts

What the mind can conceive and believe, the mind can achieve.

Napoleon Hill

The *Balanced Technology Management* concept follows the premise that an overall reduction in technology use, as well as frequent planned breaks from technology, will provide children with available time that can be spent in alternate activities. An important factor to consider is enhancing *engagement* in activity. For example, children with obesity have poor skill performance in alternate activities to technology, largely because many of them also have developmental delays. Providing increased recess time isn't enough. Children with obesity require equipment that does not challenge their physical competence. Treadmills or exercise bikes would likely prove to be more engaging for children with obesity, and should be as accessible as other playground equipment.

The actualization of *Balanced Technology Management* concepts require that adults work together to ensure children engage in the right type, duration, frequency, and intensity of activity they need to meet developmental milestones and optimize health and academic performance. The types of activity children engage in should include parameters from the *Critical Factors for Child Development* categories of movement, touch and human connection covered extensively in Section II of *Virtual Child*. Only when engagement in these activities is sufficient, is the child then allowed to access technology. There are two basic concepts to *Balanced Technology Management* theory which will be discussed extensively in below sections:

1. *What goes in = what goes out*
2. *One hour/day, day/week, week/year.*

What Goes In = What Goes Out Rule

Managing balanced use of activity and technology requires that adults adopt an "in = out" rule of whatever energy goes "into" a child's body in the form of technology, needs to be balanced by equal time spent in an energy "output" activity that optimizes that child's development. The activities chosen to balance technology's "input" can be found in the "output" categories from the *Critical Factors for Child Development* of movement, touch, or human connection. A child may be encouraged to balance television time (input) with output activities such as bike riding (movement), rough and tumble play (touch), or reading a book to their younger sibling (human connection). Other examples would be for a family to use technology for an hour after dinner, but then to come together and play a board game, wrestle or dance to music, or even clean up the house. At school, a 30 minute movie or computer work, should always be followed by 30 minutes of gym or recess time.

Why a 30 minute limit? When prototype testing the *Zone'in Program*, a program I designed to help children self regulate their energy states, we found that children started to leave *The Zone* at 30 minute durations of technology use. If a child was left continuously using technology for 45 minutes or greater, their energy was way out of *The Zone*, and was virtually impossible to "get back". *The Zone* is a termed used for a body energy state where a child is able to pay attention and learn. Energy that is either sleepy and zoned out, or charged and hyper, is not able to listen or learn. The children who used more than 30 minutes of technology did not happily transition from their technology to another activity. The children who used less than 30 minutes of technology happily transitioned to a more healthy activity.

One Hour/Day, Day/Week, Week/Year Rule

The second *Balanced Technology Management* concept is that whether children are at home, school, or in community settings, they should stop all technology use for *one hour per day, one day per week* and *one week per year*. This time off from technology allows children, families, schools and workplaces to contrast the change in their lives with and without technology use. The most important aspect to this rule, is that all family members, or school teachers and students, take the SAME time off. This allows an opportunity for relationship building and healing connections.

- **One hour per day** without technology in the home setting, might consist of the dinner hour when families work together on meal preparation and eat together around a dining room table. At school, teachers could restrict access to computers for the hour following lunch, and use lunch and recess times to promote necessary movement, touch and human connection, as well as access to nature to increase attention and learning.

- **One day per week** without technology in the home setting, might be either Saturday or Sunday when alternate activities are planned, preferably involving outdoor or nature venues. Schools could have a "Friday TECH-NO" day where technology use is restricted, and other activities are pursued such as learning to print.

- **One week per year** without technology in the home setting, could be the first week of a family holiday. Schools could designate one week during the school year where media literacy programs are enacted to raise awareness regarding technology overuse.

These aforementioned *Balanced Technology Management* principles will be applied in subsequent chapters to the six *Foundation Team* sectors, and individualized initiatives for each sector will be profiled. Readers might want to reflect on these proposed initiatives to determine whether or not they might be suitable with their own populations, and are encouraged to expand on and/or formulate their own initiatives that might more accurately reflect their own community and societal needs and goals.

Chapter 25

Measuring Success – Evidence Based Outcomes

With any home, school or community-based intervention, it is important to measure outcomes, or changes to specific areas of child performance. The following outcome measures could be tracked by an appropriate representative from the *Balanced Technology Management Foundation Team* e.g. Parent Advisory Council, teacher, principal, school-based health care team, or when available, obtained from health and education government statistics.

- **Technology reduction** – recording of total non-school related and school related technology usage for television, video games, movies, hand-held gaming devices, internet, computers, iPods, and cell phones can be collated by students, parents and schools in a simple survey method.

- **Improvements in physical health** – collation of student and teacher "sick days" away from school can be obtained from school records. Total number of medical visits by children could be monitored by parents. School, as well as health and education government statistics could be obtained regarding incidence of diagnosis of physical disorders related to sedentary lifestyle e.g. obesity, diabetes, coordination disorders, sensory processing disorders.

- **Improvements in mental health** – incidence statistics could be obtained from schools, as well as health and education governments regarding diagnosis of mental illness and psychological disorders related to technology overuse e.g. depression, anxiety, bipolar disorder, sleep impairments and subsequent prescription of psychotropic medication.

- **Improvements in behavioral health** – incidence statistics could be obtained from schools, as well as health and education governments regarding incidence of diagnosis of behavioral disorders, e.g. adhd, autism. Schools could record incidence of tantrums, self injurious acts, or other problematic behaviors.

- **Reduction in aggression** - child aggression could be monitored through school recording of student referrals to the "office", or acts of aggression against peers or teachers.

- **Improvements in student's ability to pay attention, learn and improve academic performance** – comparison of student and teacher reports regarding students ability to initiate, sustain focus on, and complete academic tasks, as well as before and after comparison of academic performance.

Measuring outcomes is not only useful to determine the effectiveness of specific *Balanced Technology Management* initiatives, but also serves to validate these interventions, and provide much needed data with which to plan future programming. The next six chapters will profile existing problems and review proposed *Balanced Technology Management* initiatives for our six target sector groups: parents, educators, health professionals, government, researchers and technology production corporations. Your

Foundation Team may wish to use these suggestions in your first meeting as a starting point to move toward formation of your own *Balanced Technology Management* initiatives for your specific community population.

Parents - The Key to Success

In the age of the "expert", parents seem to have lost their edge when it comes to being a respected authority in the life of their children. In all of my 22 years working with families, I have never seen the level of disrespect and discounting of parents by the health and education systems as I do today. Standardized testing is being performed more and more, even on children in preschools and daycares. The results of these tests are used to form elaborate diagnoses, often used then as a reason for prescribing harmful medication. The results of these assessments and accompanying diagnoses are meticulously documented in lengthy reports and presented to parents as a "true" interpretation of their child. I know this for a fact, because testing and reports is pretty much all I used to do as a school-based occupational therapist, and still do, although on a much smaller scale, today.

There will be a consequence to taking power away from parents, the most notable being the perception that the parent is no longer in charge. The parent is wrongfully led to believe they no longer understand their child, and are therefore feels as if they are unable to determine appropriate parenting rules and strategies. Parents report they feel they need to consult the "expert" before they act, because what if they were to do the "wrong" thing? By not providing parents information about the impact of technology on their child's behavior, this behavior has gone completely out of control. Instead of testing and diagnosing children, we can alternatively provide parents with information and support, empowering them to resume control over their errant and misbehaved children. Understanding their child's need for reducing technology, and increasing movement, touch and human connection, parents will get on the path toward a much healthier and happier child and family.

This section will discuss how education and health professionals can work together to put parents back in charge of raising their children, and how parents can then rightfully resume their confidence and control.

Chapter 26

Long Term Planning vs. the Quick Fix

Parents are truly the most important vehicle for change when it comes to the puzzle of technology and children, as they are the key element needed to bring children toward healthy and successful futures. The biggest impediment to parents enacting change to the ways in which their families use technology is the technology itself. The fast paced world in which we live requires that we use technology at least daily, and for some, hourly or even on a minute by minute basis. Technology production corporations are constantly marketing new and more "efficient" devices that we simply cannot live without, or so we are made to think. This immediacy with which we now live our lives has resulted in what I term "Quick Fix" parenting styles. When a child or family member has a problem, or the family as a whole has become a non-functioning unit, the quickest and shortest path is often the option chosen. While the solution might be "quick", the fix is usually "short", requiring even more drastic treatment measures down the line. Two prime examples of "quick fix" parenting with short-term outcomes are using technology to replace love and attention, and participating in behavior diagnosis and medication. "Just Say No" to technology and drugs may be difficult, but is an important first step toward a healthy and happy family life.

Balanced Technology Management Initiatives for Parents

Following are a list of possible *Balanced Technology Management* initiatives for parents, as well as a variety of useful tools to assist parents on this journey toward a new and fulfilling life.

1. **Remove all technology** from bedrooms, dining areas and cars. These are places for family conversations, which will never happen in the presence of technology.
2. **Read to your children every night** for one half hour. This could be when you get home from work, or prior to bed.
3. Do not let your children use technology for **one hour prior to bedtime**, as this will wake the area of the brain that needs to sleep.
4. **In = out**: ensure technology input = movement, touch and human connection output.
5. **One hour/day, day/week, week/year**: follow the one hour per day, one day per week, and one week per year rule of NO technology.
6. **Unplug – Don't Drug**: family trial of a 3 month period without technology prior to submitting your child for behavior diagnosis and medication.
7. **Play with your children**, help them find new interests and teach them new skills.
8. **Include grandparents** when possible in planning changes to family structure and lifestyles. They remember the joy of freedom and the value of play.
9. **Go outside**. Mother Nature is the great healer, no matter what your family issues are.

Chapter 27

Parent Tool and Repair Kits

The following tools have been used extensively by myself as parent handouts, and are designed to be effective initial first line interventions by education and health professionals to raise awareness and offer strategies to manage balanced technology use. These tools are best used in the order presented below, but can also be grouped together to be used as one handout provided during a school or community media awareness program, parent interview, or included in a school newsletter.

1. *Ten Steps to Successfully Unplug Your Child from Technology*
2. *Unplug'in Parent Brochure*
3. *Technology Schedule*
4. *Alternate Activities to Technology Use*

1. Ten Steps to Successfully Unplug Your Child from Technology

The following ten step plan was developed for parents to successfully reduce the use of technology, and start parents on the right road to begin the difficult task of managing child technology use. The *Ten Steps to Successfully Unplug Your Child from Technology* is a document designed for both the home and school based settings. *Ten Steps...* will help adults begin to negotiate the initial stages of managing balance between activities children need for growth and success with technology use.

Step One - **Become informed regarding the effects of technology on physical, mental, social and academic performance.**

Technology overuse is related to child attention problems, poor academics, aggression, family conflict, impaired sleep, developmental delays, attachment disorders, impaired body image, obesity and early sexuality. The signs of technology addiction are tolerance (need more), withdrawal (physical or mental), unintended use (didn't *mean* to use for so long), persistent desire, total time spent, displacement of other activities, and continued use (beyond what they know is good for them). The American Academy of Pediatrics recommends no technology use for 0 – 2 year olds, and no more than one to two hours per day of combined technology use, yet elementary children use on average 7.5 hours per day!

Need Help? Get informed by checking out the *Zone'in* website zonein.ca where you can read the *Zone'in Fact Sheet,* watch the *Reality Check* video clip and the *Suffer the Children* slide show, read the *Unplug – Don't Drug* policy initiative, review the research, read loads of articles, and sign up for the *Zone'in Child Development Series Newsletter.*

Step Two - Disconnect - Unplug yourself first!

As child technology use patterns parallel that of their parents, a technology addicted child is likely to live in a high technology usage household. Parents need to determine how much technology is too much, and set limits. Parents should then model balancing technology use with other activities. Schools could sponsor a *Balanced Technology Management Week* where classrooms compete to reduce technology use.

Need help? Zone'in Mixed Signals Workshop (available on live, webinar, or DVD formats) offers participants information regarding home and school *Balanced Technology Management* strategies. Schools and communities can order the *Live'in Resource Guide* for media awareness programming at www.zonein.ca.

Step Three - Reconnect - Designate "sacred time" with your children.

The root of addiction is fear of human intimacy or connection, and results from poor parent – child attachment formation. Adults may benefit from first exploring past experiences of attachment with their own parents, and think about how this experience may have affected how they relate to their own children or students. Designation of "sacred time" in the day with no technology (meals, in the car, before bedtime, and holidays) is a first start toward reconnecting with your children.

Need help? Zone'in A Cracked Foundation Workshop offers participants information regarding parent-child attachment and profiles the *Attachment Questionnaire.*

Step Four - Explore alternatives to technology as a class or family.

Not all children are interested in or value the same activities as adults, and children whose only activity is technology, have no defined skills in other activities. Fostering interest in alternative activities to technology, and learning more about individual preferences for activity, can go a long way toward promoting children's motivation to "unplug".

Need Help? Have each family member or student make a list of ten realistic, inexpensive things to do on their own, with a friend, with another family member, with a pet, indoors, and outdoors. Help children create a game, song, joke, poem, story or dance. Buy a book of games, create a story night, play wrestle, make up a silly play, build a fort of couch cushions, or doing a family cooking night are but a few of a myriad of alternatives to technology use.

Step Five - Enhance performance skills PRIOR to unplugging your children.

Children with technology addictions have poorly developed identities, social skills, relationship to nature and sense of spirit. Drastically or suddenly reducing technology with a child who has an addiction, will result in chaos at school and home, as the child is now alienated from what has become their whole meaning for living. Teachers and parents can help build performance skills by exposing children to activities that are a "just right" challenge, not too hard, not too easy.

Need help? Zone'in offers the new *Unplug'in Game* for school and home settings, a development tool to build performance skills in four dimensions: *Me, We, Nature* and *Spirit*, prior to unplugging from technology.

Step Six **- Meet developmental milestones through engagement in the three critical factors for child development - movement, touch and connection.**

Children need to rough and tumble play 2-3 hours per day, and need to spend time connecting with their parent(s), teacher and other children, in order to achieve optimal physical, mental, social and academic performance. This type of play promotes adequate sensory development of the vestibular, proprioceptive, tactile and attachment systems needed for paying attention, printing and reading.

Need help? *Zone'in Harnessing Energy* and *Back to Basics Workshops* offer participants information regarding sensory and motor development– or – buy the new *Zone'in* and *Move'in* educational programs for schools and families.

Step Seven **- Address perceptions of safety.**

Parents' perceptions of safety correlate with child time indoors in front of technology e.g. if a parent perceives the world as unsafe, that child will spend more time indoors using technology. Litigation has drastically changed playgrounds. Outdoor rough and tumble play is a biological need for children, and all children have a right to be physically active and healthy.

Need help? *Zone'in Diminishing Returns Workshop* offers participants a variety of alternative options for ensuring "safe" home and school activities to promote optimal physical and mental development, and provides the *Productivity Designs for Classroom and Gym* to improve student productivity.

Step Eight **- Create individual roles and foster inner drive.**

Children benefit from knowing their role in the big picture, and self esteem and motivation comes from being independently productive. Realistic challenges and expectations by parents and teachers, promote defined roles for children, and provide a structure and confidence where they can begin to try out new skills.

Need Help? *Zone'in Mixed Signals Workshop* offers participants the *Child Inner Drive Directive for Schools and Homes* – or – purchase the new *Unplug'in Game*.

Step Nine **- Schedule a balance between technology use and activities.**

Follow the *Zone'in Concept* of "in = out" rule where time spent using technology (energy in) should be equally balanced with time spent in movement, touch or human connection (energy out). Make up a weekly schedule with designated time for technology balanced with time for movement, touch and connection. When beginning the technology "unplug", it's important to alternate between familiar, predictable, structured activities and novel activities. The parent and teacher's job is to skillfully dance the child between predictability and novelty during the initial unplug period.

Need Help? *Zone'in Programs Inc.* offers parents, teachers and therapists' products, workshops, training and consultation to help address child technology addictions. See zonein.ca for more suggestions, or if you are a school, purchase the *Live'in Resource Guide* for media literacy programs.

Step Ten **- Link Corporations and Community to create sustainable futures for children!**

Zone'in Programs Inc. offers an invitation to all corporations involved in technology production, to direct funds back into building healthy children, schools and communities. Free recreation passes for children, building safe parks, and school camping trips are but a few sustainability initiatives to ensure children stay balanced.

Need help? *Zone'in Why Children Can't Sit Still Workshop* offers participants the *Child Development Directive* and the *Nature Directive* to optimize child health and learning. Check out zonein.ca for more information on the *Linking Corporations to Community Initiative.*

2. Unplug'in Parent Brochure

"Must read" information for everyone who loves their children.

The following information is compiled from the *Unplug'in Parent Brochure* available on the *Zone'in* website www.zonein.ca. This information could be useful for parents groups, education and health professionals who would like to formulate brochures or handouts for parents to raise information regarding the harmful effects of technology on their children.

Technology Facts

- **FACT** - The average child spends 7.5 hours per day watching television, playing video games, using the internet or talking/texting on their cell phone.
- **FACT** - 75% of North American children have some form of technology (computer, television, video games) in their bedrooms.
- **FACT** - The average parent spends 3.5 minutes in meaningful conversation with their child – PER WEEK.
- **FACT** - Active Healthy Kids Canada report gave Canadian children a grade "D" for physical activity.
- **FACT** - In order for children to develop properly, they require lots of movement, touch and connection with their friends and family members.
- **FACT** - Television, video game and internet overuse is linked to aggression, developmental delays, impaired health, obesity, poor body image, addictions to drugs/alcohol/cigarettes, attention problems, trouble sleeping, poor school performance, family conflicts, and early sexual experiences.
- **FACT** - Childhood diagnosis of mental disorders has tripled in the past five years, with 15% of children diagnosed with a mental illness.
- **FACT** - Prescription of psychotrophic (mind altering) medication to toddlers 2 – 4 years of age has tripled in the past five years.
- **FACT** - Only 30% of parents set rules for their children restricting technology use. Those children whose parents impose technology restrictions, use 30% less technology.

Research references are available on *Zone'in Fact Sheet* at zonein.ca.

How do you know if your child is addicted to technology?

- Do you have a hard time prying your child away from technology including television, video games, internet or cell phones?

178

- Does your child's behavior change following prolonged use of technology?
- Has your child gone all day without eating, because he/she is glued to technology?
- Does your child watch the same amount of television, or play the same amount of video games as they used to, but does not appear to get the same level of satisfaction as they used to?
- Can your child imagine life without technology? What else would they do?
- Does your child ever use more technology for longer than they intended, or longer than you allowed?
- Have you ever tried to stop your child from using technology, but couldn't?
- Does technology take up all of your child's free time?
- Does your child sometimes use technology, when they should be spending time with family or friends, doing homework, or going to bed?
- Does your child continue to use technology, even though they know it isn't good for them?

If you answered 'yes' to three or more of the questions above, based on the medical definition of "addiction" your child is addicted to technology.

What does this mean for your family?

Chances are if your child or entire family is addicted to technology, your lives have been dramatically affected. Short tempers, rude comments, angry outbursts, no energy to do any household chores or outdoor play, are common in families with television, video game or internet addictions.

Children with technology addictions often disconnect from themselves, others and nature. They may exhibit behavior problems, not know how to interact with other children, or may seem either withdrawn or hyperactive. Children with technology addictions also may have difficulty paying attention at school. Families with technology addictions may have difficulties interacting and connecting with each other in a healthy way, and may be prone to intense conflict.

How does this affect your child in the classroom?

For every one hour of television, video games and internet your child uses per day, they will have a 10% chance of an attention problem by age seven. So if your child uses 7.5 hours of technology per day, they will have a 75% chance of having attention problems.

Ability to pay attention is essential for academic performance. If your child has a TV in their bedroom, chances are they will also be sleep deprived at school, further limiting their ability to perform academically. Children's bodies need to move to learn. When children sit in front of a screen, they are not moving, and their body energy becomes either zoned out or hyper. When children's bodies move, their body energy becomes balanced, and learning is easy.

What can you do now?

Children need to *learn* how to play, and parents need to teach them. Instead of trying to DO something to your children, try to BE something to them. Your children would rather have you play with them any day, than watch television or play video games. The activities listed below will encourage family re-connection and prove to be fun for all. Your child will love you for taking the time to engage in activities with them, instead of popping in a movie "babysitter".

Ride bikes
Build a couch or table fort
Eat dinner as a family
Be artistic – paint, color, make crafts
Dance
Play wrestle
Listen to music
Play cards
Play a board game
Invent your own game
Garden or together
Read a book
Play a sport
Cook a meal together
Do chores together

Family life can be busy, and it may be hard to find time to spend with your children. After work, dinner needs cooking, and houses need cleaning. Why not get your kids to help you with these chores? You'd be surprised at how happy your child can be cutting vegetables while chatting with mom and dad.

Families that play together stay together!

3. Technology Schedule

The *Technology Schedule* is a tool I designed for parents and teachers to help children manage balance between activities required for growth and success, with technology use. Managing balance between technology use and movement, touch and human connection, is essential for development of child physical, mental, social and academic ability.

The *Technology Schedule* is designed to be attached to a child's fridge at home, or used in a binder at school. The schedule requires that on Sunday nights, children schedule their 1-2 hours per week of technology use, as well as schedule the equivalent amount of movement, touch and human connection activities (example listed on schedule). This time of scheduling of technology and activities could be used as a negotiation time between parents and children regarding types of acceptable television programs, video games, movies and internet usage. Some children will require parent or teacher assistance to identify desirable activities that are not related to technology.

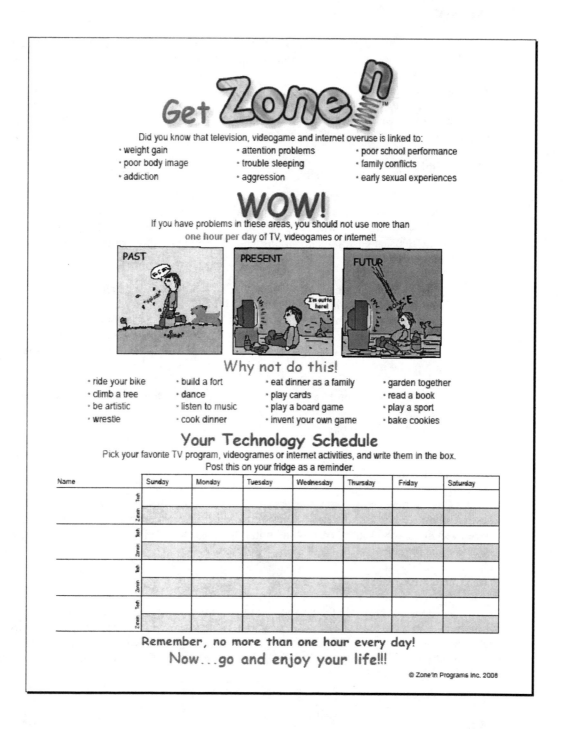

4. Alternative Activities to Technology Use

By Yourself

Read a book, play a card game, play a board game, sing like no one is listening, dance like no one is watching, cook something good, tickle yourself, give yourself a nice ear and face massage, do sit/push ups, run in place like someone is chasing you, plant something, watch the clouds/stars, breathe like you can't get enough, draw pictures no one can understand, write a goofy story, make up silly jokes, look at yourself in the mirror and smile, make flash cards with useless information on them, make a fort out of couch cushions, take your dog for a walk, scribble all over the phone book.

With a Friend

Indoors: play clapping/rhyming games, play "rock, paper, scissors", play "I spy with my little eye", play "vegetable-plant-mineral", make cookies, play board games, make up a silly card game, dye eggs when it's not Easter, dress up when it's not Halloween, make scary faces and unusual noises, make an obstacle course out of your parents furniture, dress up in your parents clothes.

Outdoors Summer: play tag, play capture the flag, ride a bike, climb a tree, make a fort out of cardboard scraps, do silly dog and cat imitations, wash your dog, make a water slide, wash your Mom's car, make a city with sticks and leaves, damn running water with pebbles, dig holes in the dirt and bury stuff, make a rope swing in a tree, swing from a tree branch, sled down grassy hills on pieces of cardboard, clean up the yard, make a pile of leaves and jump into it.

Outdoors Winter: build a fort out of snow, build a snow (wo)man, squirt colored water on the snow and make pictures, slide down snowy hills on pieces of cardboard or plastic garbage bags, skate on the ice with slippery shoes, play ice hockey with brooms and a tennis ball.

With Your Family

Cook a new and strange dinner every week, have movie night with popcorn, play wrestle, pillow fights before bed, read to your younger sibling, do a family drama night where everyone plays each other, tell one good thing and one bad thing that happened each day at the dinner table.

With Your Classroom

Make up a classroom theme song, make up a rap dance, have classroom square ball competitions at recess, dress like the teachers, switch gender dress up day, pajama day, shake and wiggle time every 20 minutes, go outside as a class as often as you can, make up a play and act it out for the school, rotating DJ for regular classroom music time.

Educators - Evidence Based Research

A Student's Concerns

Our generation has been exposed to the media way too early. I think that's degrading society to the point that we're not going to be able to recover. Technology is great, but we don't need it.

I think we're addicted to needing to have new messages. We feel needed, and we're almost addicted to that feeling.

You don't have to go live in the woods, but you have to be conscious about how you use these devices.

I think it's easier to think about how technology is a factor in our lives when we step out of it.

Grade 11 students from Lincoln High School in Portland, Oregon, following a four day technology "unplug".

A frequent question I ask children is "why do you go to school"? Most children respond with the answer "to learn". When I follow with the question "learn what?" many children either say they "don't know", or they say they have to learn "stuff" to get a job. The apparent confusion children have regarding why they are at school, should act as a huge wake up call to educators. Children no longer go to school to learn "the basics" of printing and reading, nor do they go to school to socialize with their peers. Schools of today have changed dramatically over the past decade, so much so that children no longer even know why they are there. Gone are the chalk boards that used to fill at least 3 of the 4 walls, a place where children used to stand while learning to print. Gone are the shelves of text books, the counters full of science experiments, the walls full of art work. Printing is now considered antiquated in the education system, as is the reading of books. Science, socials, math, and even art and music, now often have computer based curriculum.

The whole education system appears to be under the illusion that computers can actually teach children just about everything, and even for some subjects actually replace the teacher, but at what long term costs to the student? This illusion that technology can teach children literacy not only lacks any research evidence, but also just doesn't make sense. Teachers still assign grades to children based on work they produce using pencil and paper. Yet - teachers have quit teaching children to print. At the possible expense of creating a whole generation of illiterate adults, where is the evidence to support these short-sighted and prevalent trends to increase the use of computers in the education system?

Chapter 28

Learning Disability or Teaching Disability?

A Teacher's Concerns

Having taught in various parts of North America, I observed cultural differences in the areas that I worked. In Guadalajara, Mexico, during the late 1980's, technology was not a prevalent concern regarding monopolization of students' time and attention. Having taught for two years in Coral Harbour, Nunavut, Canada from 1988-1990, the Inuit children had other concerns than being engrossed with technology...as we were in a very remote settlement in the middle of Hudson's Bay.

Finally having spent the bulk of my teaching time on the Sunshine Coast of British Columbia, Canada I noticed over the years how the students became more and more engaged with technology as it became much more available. Parents used to ask me how I was going to help them stop their children from watching so much t.v.?! I suggested that they simply turn the t.v. off and was met with incredulity. I mentioned that a t.v. in the bedroom was not a good idea as it made it too easy to be engulfed by the programs and difficult for the parents to monitor what was being watched. I also stressed how so much t.v. watching took away their study time.

With the prevalence of games, cell phones etc I witnessed students being more focused to being easily distracted and constantly bombarded with interruptions.

A sense of 'entitlement' by the students, knowing that they could access whatever they wanted, when they wanted, seemed to have shifted the focus from 'self-starter' and 'self-motivated' to getting what they wanted technologically without having to work for it.

Students mimicking what they experienced through the content of the video games, was probably the most disturbing. There was this disengagement with the 'feelings' of what was going on in real life since the games seemed to have de-sensitized them. A hurt child on the playground seemed 'unreal' like in the games where the player gets back up and does it again.

Bet Diening-Weatherston, parent of two teenaged boys, former elementary school teacher and current *Journey Practitioner* and *Coach.*

The second most important person in a child's life is their teacher. In a child's school lifetime, they will spend 1200 hours per year with each teacher, totaling 14,400 hours spent in school during their elementary, middle and high school grades. This time spent in school should be optimized for learning useful concepts and enhancing literacy necessary for eventual employment, not plugging children into computers and hope that by some fluke they actually will absorb something useful. Unfortunately the extent of developmental delay in today's classrooms has created a significant "gap" in student ability level. Instead of teaching to developmental level, teachers continue to teach grade specific material, advancing ill prepared students through the grades regardless of their performance.

Resulting frustration and behavior in students is creating classrooms that are nightmares for teachers and students alike. So, do we really have a situation of increasing levels of learning disabled children, or have teachers become "disabled" by a system that has forgotten the importance of teaching the basics?

It almost seems as if teaching "the basics" is no longer of value to education governments, who have diluted the basics with a host of new, yet untested computerized curriculum. What happens when whole systems throw out the "old" to make way for the "new"? With rapidly evolving computer technologies, it is logistically impossible for schools to provide students with instruction in the 3 R's (reading, writing and arithmetic), as well as provide up to date instruction in computer technologies. Costs associated with provision of up to date technology will require diversion of funds from other areas. Where else can an already diminished budget be diminished further?

As children are now exposed to an average 7.5 hours per day of entertainment technology in the home, and 6.5 hours per day in schools (who use wireless internet), there are many technology reduction initiatives that can be immediately implemented in school settings to begin to address safety issues inherent with the rampant overuse of technology by children. Schools need to first ensure that they are creating environments that promote healthy development and optimal attention and learning. We learned in Section I that wireless internet emits potentially harmful low frequency electromagnetic radiation, which in cell phones has been associated with brain cancer (Khurara, 2009). I was recently told by teachers that the British Columbia Education Ministry is encouraging the placement of computers in kindergarten classrooms for pre-reading skill training. This initiative not only lacks supporting evidence, but based on current research, will likely result in irreversible long term harm to child health.

Balanced Technology Management Initiatives for Educators

While the implications of this research are far reaching and nothing short of profound, more research needs to be generated to validate and replicate these findings in order to provide informed guidelines for technology use restrictions. In the meanwhile, to sit and do nothing will most likely prove harmful to children. When in doubt, erring on the side of caution is a wise guideline to follow. But how cautious should we be, and should we be more cautious with young children, than adolescents and high school age? There are many technology reduction initiatives that can be immediately implemented in homes, schools and community settings to begin to address safety issues inherent with the rampant overuse of technology by children. The following suggestions could be a place to start for *Balanced Technology Management Foundation Teams* discussions with their respective technology school-based teams.

1. **Reduce overall technology use** to expert recommendations from the American Academy of Pediatrics and the Canadian Pediatric Society to 1-2 hours per day. As home technology use by children averages 7.5 hours per day, extraordinary efforts need to be enacted by education and professionals to achieve these significantly reduced levels.
2. **Establish risk/harm reduction policies for staff and students regarding technology use**. These policies should take into account that children with photophobic conditions such as autism are at risk for seizures.
3. **Restrict all school technologies from children younger than grade six**, with the exception of children who require technology to access curriculum due to a physical disability. Schools eliminating technology use for children younger than grade six would make a tremendous difference in overall technology use, and send a message home to parents regarding the inherent dangers associated with technology use. Health and education governments need support this initiative, as

they are presently recommending use of computers in kindergarten.

4. **Prohibit entertainment technology use AT ALL TIMES in school settings**. Children are already using 7.5 hours per day at home, so don't allow additional use at school.

5. **Return to the use of cable based internet** is one way to reduce radiation from electromagnetic fields, as wireless internet emits higher levels of EMF as they have to "search" for a signal.

6. **Only use technology products that are evidenced based** and without conflict of interest e.g. research that was not conducted by the technology production company.

7. **Stop use of all cell phones with children younger than grade eight**, and create safe distances between cell phone and the brain in adolescents through mandatory use of remote devices e.g. Blue Tooth console bluetooth.com. Five years ago children did not have cell phones. They don't need them now.

8. **Redirect education focus onto literacy enhancing initiatives** e.g. teach printing and reading. Universities who offer educator training should instruct new teachers in the use of "tried and true" methods for teaching children how to print. *The MacLean's Method* was a proven "strategy-based" technique successful in achieving printing literacy for several decades. Education governments should provide curriculum-based guidelines for not only printing instruction, but also evaluation methods, to improve on teacher consistency regarding printing.

Even when provided with all this information about the detrimental effects of technology on children, few brave individuals in school-based settings are willing to walk the path toward technology management. Frequently, I hear from my workshop participants that there is no one to form a potential *Balanced Technology Management Foundation Team* with! From education government, right down to the janitorial staff, everyone seems to be on the "technology train." I always respond with encouragement for teachers to ask the question "Show me the evidence." Demanding to see unbiased research evidence for inclusion of computer technology in the education arena, should raise a few eyebrows, and shed some light on what is currently a very dark subject.

Chapter 29

Increasing Profits in the Classroom – Proven Tools for Success

To increase profits in the classroom, educators need to redefine the ways in which children learn. Learning is best optimized through use of movement, touch, human connection and access to nature, and balancing those activities with technology. In order to help schools work toward *Balanced Technology Management* and academic success, I've designed the following useful tools for the education community. Each of these tools will be described in length, with references made for additional resource materials. I suggest your *Foundation Team* review these tools to determine if they would be suitable for your environment or school. Identification of other useful tools and techniques may result from the process of learning about the details of my suggestions and recommendations.

1. **Zone'in Program** – improves sensory processing, self regulation and attention.
2. **Zone'in Stations for Classroom and Gym** – school application of the *Zone'in Program*
3. **Move'in Program** – assesses developmental level and improves printing and reading skill.
4. **Unplug'in Program** – builds confidence and skills in activities alternate to technology.
5. **Live'in Resource Guide** – media literacy program to manage balanced technology use in homes, schools and in communities.
6. **Foundation Series Workshops** – six seminars to improve knowledge regarding sensory, motor, attachment, technology, optimal learning, and school design for success.
7. **Instructor Training** – certification course to qualify occupational therapists to perform *Foundation Series Workshops*.

The Zone'in Program

While working with children in school settings, I often observed that learning difficulties weren't necessarily relevant to a child's intelligence, but more relevant to that child's ability to stay focused and alert. This observation resulted in the development of a program called "Zone'in" which enables a child to self regulate their energy, and use a variety of tools and techniques to get their energy *Zone'in to Learn*. A child who is not alert at all, or is hyper vigilant and *too* alert, is unable to register and make sense of incoming information necessary to learn. What teachers and parents often forget is that the origin for learning and attention is located in the body, not the brain. When a child's body energy is *grounded* and *centered*, then their brain is "primed" to operate efficiently and effectively.

Children ground their energy through engaging their bodies in specific types of movement, mainly the type of movement we use when doing *heavy work* activities involving resistive or isometric actions. Pushing or pulling against a resistance allows a release of pent up body energy, calming and centering the child's body, and promoting optimal attention and learning. Children therefore need to move to learn, and when children don't move, their energy is all over the map, and learning is impossible. Teachers and parents can no more tell a child to sit still and pay attention than they can stop a bee from flying. Just as bees are designed to fly, children's bodies are designed to move. When children don't move, the result is impairments to their physical, mental, social and academic systems.

During in-classroom prototype testing of the *Zone'in Program*, a programs for children ages 5 – 12 years of age, we found that specific types of sensation and movement optimized children's attention and learning, whereas other types either made no difference or were detrimental to children's overall academic performance. We also discovered through trials of numerous sensory and motor tools and techniques, that each child's arousal system is unique, precluding use of whole-classroom type activities. Children whose energy was in the *Zone* already, who then used a *Zone'in* tool or technique during whole-classroom testing, were quite upset when they found their energy had shifted to either too charged or too hyper, thus disabling their learning. Each child has the right to be provided with information and an opportunity to develop their own specific activities to regulate their sensory system body energy. Achieving optimal arousal state for attention and learning can be achieved through use of the widely popular *Zone'in Program* which comes with *Zone-O-Meters* to measure energy, as well as the fun *Zone'in DVD*, *Know Your Zone* and *Tone Your Zone* posters and a variety of *Zone'in* sensory and motor tools and techniques to get while classrooms *Zone'in to* *Learn!*

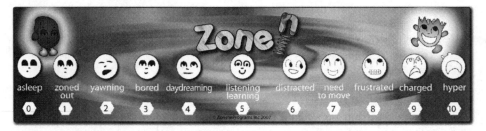

Highly anxious or alternatively depressed children often have trouble even getting themselves to school, much less paying attention and learning. The energy states of these children are either through the roof (anxious) or utterly depleted (depressed), neither of which is optimal for school work. These children may oscillate from anxious to depressed and back again in very short time frames, a phenomenon that contributes to the rising incidence of what is commonly termed "bipolar disorder". In *Zone'in* terminology, these children with bipolar diagnoses have energy that is "way out of the *Zone*", fluctuating between sleepy and zoned out to hyper and charged, as depicted in below *Zone-O-Meter* graphic. These children require intense and continuous sensory and motor interventions to bring them back and keep them in the *Zone* to learn. The *Zone'in* model is a "concentric" as opposed to a "linear" model, and explains why some children would report their energy state is a 4 (daydreaming) *and* a 6 (distracted), or a 2 (yawning) *and* an 8 (frustrated), *at the same time*. When children's "mood" state is described to them as an "energy" state, and they are provided with sensory and motor tools and techniques to change their energy, their life is simplified. Offering children the opportunity to self regulate their energy states, as opposed to medicating them, would be an long term "fix", one that is so much safer and healthier than medication.

Creating *Zone'in* Stations in Classrooms and Gyms

Requirements

Creating *Zone'in Stations* require parents and/or school staff use the *Zone'in Program* (or another program that promotes self regulation) to help children self regulate their energy bodies to optimize attention and learning.

Concept

Zone'in classroom and gym stations should encompass the *Zone'in Concept* which states the following:

- *Children need to move to learn* – at least 2-3 hours per day rough and tumble play is require for optimal sensory and motor development and subsequent learning.
- *Energy in = energy out* - children require breaks AT LEAST every 20 minutes to get their energy *Zone'in to Learn.*
- *Children know what they need* – and meeting these needs will result in achieving an optimal attention state. Children should be provided with the opportunity to choose what, when and how long they do a *Zone'in* technique or use a *Zone'in* tool.

Materials

Refer to the *Zone'in Program* and the *Zone'in Recommended Tools and Techniques* form. Many of these tools can be fabricated or attained through local suppliers for free, so suggestion would be to start cheap, and once you see the results, go to local funding groups, or apply to technology production corporations for the more expensive items.

Classrooms

Refer to the following *Zone'in to Learn – Classroom Design* handout. Work with the students to determine two locations (corners) in classroom to create the *Zone'in Cave* and *Gas Station*. This space can be as small as a 5' X 5' area, preferably designated by a square of carpet to stabilize items. Creating the *Zone'in Cave* could be as simple as moving a book shelf away from the wall to create space behind, and anchoring a blanket to create a "womb space". The *Gas Station* could be a simple chin up bar, or rusty exercise bike (high resistance).

Gyms

Refer to the *Zone'in to Learn – Gym Design* handout. Gyms should be open before school, during recess, lunch and after school to allow necessary "energy out" and rough and tumble play. There is no end to the variety of tools and techniques that can be used to optimize energy, but schools will want to focus on students achieving lots of proprioceptive (push, pull, lift, carry), vestibular (swinging/spinning) and tactile (deep pressure wrapping) sensory stimulation for optimal attention to learn.

Zone'in to Learn
Classroom Design

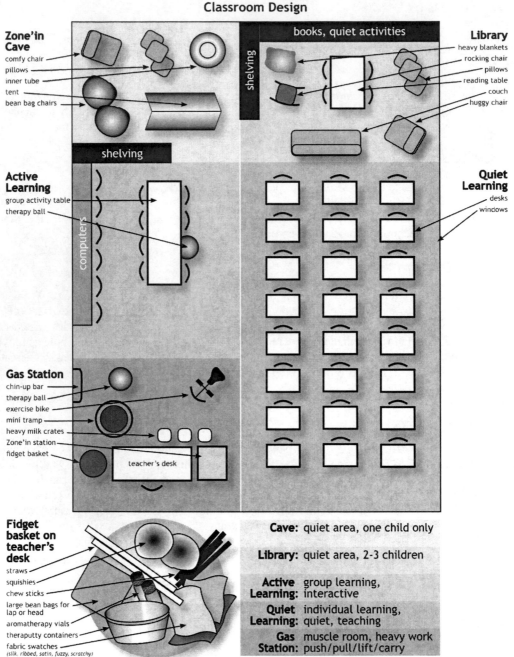

Zone'in Cave
- comfy chair
- pillows
- inner tube
- tent
- bean bag chairs

books, quiet activities

shelving

Library
- heavy blankets
- rocking chair
- pillows
- reading table
- couch
- huggy chair

shelving

Active Learning
- group activity table
- therapy ball

computers

Quiet Learning
- desks
- windows

Gas Station
- chin-up bar
- therapy ball
- exercise bike
- mini tramp
- heavy milk crates
- Zone'in station
- fidget basket

teacher's desk

Fidget basket on teacher's desk
- straws
- squishies
- chew sticks
- large bean bags for lap or head
- aromatherapy vials
- theraputty containers
- fabric swatches *(silk, ribbed, satin, fuzzy, scratchy)*

Cave:	quiet area, one child only
Library:	quiet area, 2-3 children
Active Learning:	group learning, interactive
Quiet Learning:	individual learning, quiet, teaching
Gas Station:	muscle room, heavy work push/pull/lift/carry

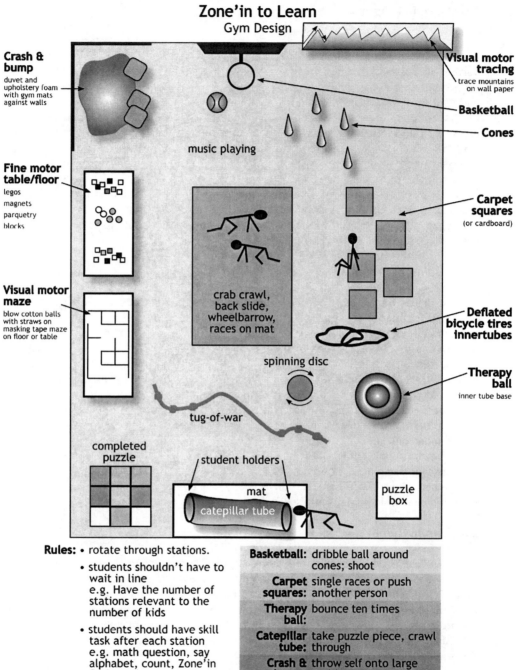

Zone'in to Learn
Gym Design

Crash & bump
duvet and upholstery foam with gym mats against walls

Fine motor table/floor
legos
magnets
parquetry
blocks

Visual motor maze
blow cotton balls with straws on masking tape maze on floor or table

music playing

crab crawl, back slide, wheelbarrow, races on mat

spinning disc

tug-of-war

completed puzzle

student holders

catepillar tube

mat

puzzle box

Visual motor tracing
trace mountains on wall paper

Basketball

Cones

Carpet squares
(or cardboard)

Deflated bicycle tires innertubes

Therapy ball
inner tube base

Rules:
- rotate through stations.
- students shouldn't have to wait in line
  e.g. Have the number of stations relevant to the number of kids
- students should have skill task after each station
  e.g. math question, say alphabet, count, Zone'in flash cards

Basketball:	dribble ball around cones; shoot
Carpet squares:	single races or push another person
Therapy ball:	bounce ten times
Catepillar tube:	take puzzle piece, crawl through
Crash & bump:	throw self onto large cushion

The Move'in Program

The *Move'in Program* is an individualized assessment and intervention to improve printing and reading skill in the form of a game board, DVD, computer program and a variety of tools and techniques. The *Move'in Program* is for children ages 5-12, and can be implemented in home, clinic or classroom based settings. Children form into groups of four and as they watch an instructional DVD, they "play" the *Ready, Set, Move'in* game which takes them on a fun and informative "printing adventure". Each of the 13 game squares is an aspect of fine motor skill necessary for optimal performance in printing and reading. The DVD shows children a task to perform, and if they have trouble, shows them what they need to do to improve their skill. When children are finished playing the game, they take the results down to the computer lab to enter them onto a computer which is connected to the internet (as opposed to wireless). The *Play'in the Lines* computer program in addition to data basing each child's performance, allows the children to print off customized journal and worksheets, as well as shows them how to make all the strokes, shapes, capital and small case letters, and numbers.

The Unplug'in Program

The *Unplug'in Program* is designed to build confidence and performance in activities alternate to technology, so children can become aware of why they use technology, and ultimately reduce their reliance and use. In the form of a game board and cards, children travel through the four dimensions of *Me, We, Spirit* and *Nature* forming relationships with themselves, others, their spirit self and mother nature. When playing the *Unplug'in* game, children travel between dimensions through use of *Journey Cards* which promote creativity and imagination. *To Do Cards* offer fun and silly activities, *Unplug'in Cards* raise awareness regarding technology use, and *What If Cards* build problem solving skill. By the time children reach the Unplug'in Victory Mile, they have explored numerous aspects of the four dimensions, and discovered a variety of alternate activities to technology use. Whether played with friends, family or classmates, children learn how to navigate their way out of the "technology trap" and are on their way toward a life of balancing activities with technology use. When played with parents, conversation can proceed toward a family discussion to determine technology limits and schedules.

The Live'in Resource Guide

The *Live'in Resource Guide* is a media literacy program manual, designed to be used in conjunction with information from the *Virtual Child* book. *Live'in* can be used in home, school and community settings, and contains teacher modules that help elementary aged children identify the role of technology in their lives though a series of home or classroom-based exercises. *Live'in* also contains a variety of tools and techniques for schools to use to implement programs that manage balance between activities children need for growth and success with technology use.

Foundation Series Workshops

Zone'in Programs Inc. offers both a workshop and consultative service model to education and health professionals. These services assist the professionals to better understand the impact of technology on the developing child, and enhance child development and academic performance. When a child's sensory and motor processing improve, so does their attention, literacy and classroom behavior. *Zone'in Programs Inc.*

offers the following half day workshops for education and health professionals called *The Foundation Series*, available in live, webinar and DVD formats. *The Foundation Series* covers the following six topic areas to provide the latest research and techniques to assess and treat the 21st century technology addicted, developmentally delayed child.

1. **Sensory Processing** – covers sensory integration and self regulation theory, three critical factors for child development of touch, movement and human connection, application of the *Sensory Observations and Strategies* form, and profiles the *Zone'in Program* and other interventions to improve sensory processing and attention.

2. **Motor Development** – addresses the impact of a decline in printing instruction on literacy, profiles current research regarding literacy, application of the *Fine Motor Observations and Strategies* form, and profiles the *Move'in Program* and other interventions that improve printing.

3. **Attachment and Addictions** – profiles research that show how addictions and mental illness result from dysfunctional attachments, and proposes inclusion of treatment by health professionals to address parent/child attachment development.

4. **Technology Overuse** – profiles research on the impact of technology on child physical, mental, social and academic performance and recommends interventions that promote activities children need for growth and success.

5. **Science of Attention and Learning** – neurobiology of why children need to move to learn, profiles impact of nature as an attention-restorative agent, instructs how to implement touch, movement and human connection strategies in home, school, clinic and community settings.

6. **Classroom, Gym and Playground Design for Success** – covers why schools are struggling with the "gap" and how to increase returns on investment through re-designing environments for student productivity.

Instructor Training Program

In order to pass along this information in a timely manner by qualified health professionals, I have developed the *Zone'in Instructor Training Program* for certified occupational therapists. A one week training module provides *Level One Instructor Status* which allows instructors to administer *Foundation Series Workshops* in their own communities. Application procedures are available on the *Zone'in* website zonein.ca.

Chapter 30

Managing Difficult Child Behavior

Managing child behavior in school settings poses potential injury risk, to both staff and students, resulting in increased use of questionable practices. In the past decade, schools have witnessed an unprecedented rise in the use of various forms of restraint to control child behavior: medication of children, use of seclusion rooms, and physical restraint. To protect children and staff, it is imperative that schools take proactive measures to establish effective child behavior interventions and policies that consistently emphasize eliminating seclusion and restraints. This section contrasts the high risk and cost of this behavior management method to the low risk and cost of improving access to green space and movement.

Schools Operating Safely (SOS) – Child Behavior Management Policy and Procedures
Ten Alternatives to Use of Psychotropic Medication, Seclusion, and Restraints

The following ten evidenced based interventions are recommended for school implementation for a six month period, prior to student behavioral diagnosis, medication, or use of seclusion rooms or restraints. *Schools Operating Safely* can be used by school administrations as a guideline to determine proactive interventions to manage escalating child behaviors that would reduce risk or injury to students and staff. Potential funding for SOS equipment can be obtained through applications to pharmaceutical and/or technology production corporations. Implementation of the SOS policy should not only reduce risk of injury to students and staff, but also will serve to improve student's physical, mental, social and academic performance. Therefore, school measurement of the following outcomes are suggested, following a gathering of baseline data on the following: attention and learning ability, printing output speed, obesity, developmental delay, behavior, office referrals, school fights, suspensions and grades. Please refer to *Zone'in Fact Sheet* available on *Zone'in* website zonein.ca for a comprehensive research referenced facts to support this initiative.

Schools Operating Safely (SOS) - Policy and Procedures	Equipment Required	Projected Date
1. No Restraints		
No behavior diagnosis, medication, use of seclusion or restraints for six month period *(Breggin, 2009)*. Consider introduction of this policy at your next staff meeting or student Individual Education Plan.		
2. Limit Technology		
No technology use during breaks or recess *(Small, 2008)*. All children should be outside, restricting ALL hand held devices e.g. cell phones, iPods, electronic games.		
3. Physical Exercise		
45 minutes per day cardiovascular exercise *(Ratey, 2009)*. Add treadmills, exercise bikes, stationary weight sets, mini trampolines, wobble boards, and chin-up bars to classrooms, gym or hallways.		
4. Access Nature		
20 minutes per day access to "green space" *(Faber-Taylor, 2001)*. Nature is attention-restorative, so teach one subject per day outdoor; create "green space" by planting trees, grass, gardens, and shrubs.		
5. Take Breaks		
Unrestricted breaks - fresh air, bathroom, standing desk, Zone'in Tools and Techniques *(Rowan, 2005). Establish Zone'in Stations in every classroom with designated rules and procedures.*		
6. Organize Activities		
Physical Education Instructors for organized recess and gym activities (Pelligrini, 2005). Designate one teacher for planning organized gym activities before/after school, recess and lunch time inter-murals, sports coaching etc.		
7. Improve Playgrounds		
Access to "sensational" playgrounds – vestibular, tactile, proprioceptive input (Ayers, 1979). Minimize injury risk and maximize attaining critical factors for child growth and academic success through use of equipment that is suspended and promotes "heavy work".		
8. Teach Printing		
45 minutes per day printing instruction (Graham, 2008). Children who can't print, yet are required to do so on a daily basis, hate school. Use consistent printing strategy instruction and evaluation for 4-5 ten minute periods per day. Every child has the right to learn to print.		
9. Build Attachment		
Build respectful student-teacher connection and attachment (Bowlby, 1990). Children with difficult behaviors often have difficult families, necessitating forming healthy connections with teachers, support staff, and older students. Eye contact, empathetic listening, and appropriate touch build attachment.		
10. Educate Parents		
Parent education - limit combined technology use to 1-2 hours per day (AAP, 2004). Yearly *Balanced Technology Management* modules (*Live'in Resource Guide)* offer students and parents accurate information and strategies; hand out family *Technology Screens* at parent-teacher meetings.		

Health Professionals - A Diagnostic Crisis

The Lonely Life of the Hospital Volunteer

Volunteers in hospitals and health facilities are getting very little business due to electronic options that patients now have.

Good people who have found time in their week to volunteer are often waiting alone in playrooms without customers, or declined as company wherever patients prefer their electronic games, video options or cell phones. Unfortunately electronic alternatives are now the preference for a good chunk of the patient population and volunteers are spending more and more time cleaning things and waiting for patients who seldom partake in their services.

Steve Brosnihan, Resident Cartoonist, Children's Hospital, Road Island

There isn't a health professional out there that hasn't been hit hard by the impact of technology overuse by children. Whether in the medical, rehabilitative, psychology or psychiatry field, many of the presenting problems of today's children are either caused by, or associated with high levels of technology use. As health professionals strive to stay abreast of all the new research, and determine how to treat the shear volume of children presenting with physical, mental, social and academic impairments, the health system appears to be wholly inadequate and unprepared to deal with this onslaught. The health care system requires, at the very least, an extensive review of existing research to guide best practices toward an ethical treatment of children. To continue to participate in the prolific diagnosis and medication of children who may have technology addictions, and not offering healthy alternatives, is not in the best interests of anyone.

Chapter 31

One Nation NOT Under Therapy

The first step for health care systems to take would be to understand the impact of technology on the developing child and their family structure. The next step is for health care systems would be to enact management initiatives to ensure children balance participation in activities that help them grow and succeed, with their use of technology. Health professionals can investigate and examine the extent of technology overuse and addictions through the routine use of the *Technology Screen* and *Technology Guideline* tools previously detailed and provided for readers in Section I. After this information is collated and analyzed, health care systems will then be able to determine further appropriate interventions and treatments for these children.

Some potential problem areas for consideration by health professionals are listed below, and can be used as a template for further discussion at *Foundation Team* meetings. This list is just a few of the questions being asked by parents, teachers, health professionals, government, and researchers not only in North America, but on a world stage.

Developmental Delay: how can a limited supply of health care professionals assess and treat the rising incidence of 30% developmental delay at school entry? Should individualized models be replaced by full class assessment and intervention techniques?

Mental Illness and Behavior Management: how can health care professionals address the rising incidence of 15% mental illness in elementary children, in addition to rising levels of aggression and behavior management difficulties? What is the role of the health care professional in the escalation of behavior diagnosis and use of psychotropic medication?

Sensory Overload: how much technology is too much, and should child care clinics allow access to entertainment technology? Does the overuse of technology cause auditory and visual sensory impairment, and to what extent is *Sensory Processing Disorder* related to technology overuse? Do children with autism have an increased risk of seizure activity with video game use?

Poor Attention: how can clinicians facilitate optimal attention span of children who are sensory and sleep deprived from overuse of technology in both clinic and home settings?

Sedentary Lifestyle: how can clinicians promote essential movement at home and in community, as well as make recommendations for classroom, gym and playground schools settings?

Empirical Evidence: when there is little or no research to support the use of computers in school settings, and is it the responsibility of the health care professional to provide consultation regarding state of the art computers for children with mild cognitive, sensory or motor based disorders?

TeleHealth: to what extent should the use of remote imaging be used by health professionals in the assessment and treatment of children as a time or cost saving measure?

Balanced Technology Management Initiatives for Health Professionals

The following *Balanced Technology Management* initiatives will offer the health care professional a guide toward improving their quality of service to children.

1. Routine use of the *Technology Screen* and *Technology Guidelines* in the assessment and intervention process for all children.
2. Provide parents with *accurate, research-based, appropriate information* regarding the impact of technology on children, and how to manage balance between activities children need for growth and success and technology. This information can be passed directly to parents by clinicians, or community awareness campaigns through local health units e.g. posters, brochures, handouts.
3. *Restrict* all technology from *daycare* and *pre-school* settings.
4. *Unplug – Don't Drug Policy*: mandatory 3 month family technology "unplug" trial prior to behavior diagnosis and medication.
5. *Limit TeleHealth* with children until sufficient research supports its use.

Unplug - Don't Drug Policy

Whether you are a parent, teacher, therapist, social worker, physician, pediatrician, psychologist or psychiatrist, adopting a cautious approach to child behavior diagnosis and medication is imperative if we are to ensure sustainable futures for our children. Preliminary steps toward addressing problem behaviors in children should mandate parental involvement, as children are a product of their environments. All intervention plans and recommendations should contain both home and school-based initiatives, and be team based consisting of input from a variety of professionals.

As technology overuse is causally linked to problematic behaviors in children, as well as to a variety of mental illnesses, managing technology reduction or elimination should be every education and health professional's first step in child behavior management. As child technology use patterns follow that of their parents, a technology "unplug" trial by the whole family would be warranted prior to investing any further time on costly diagnosis and potentially harmful medication. Following use of the *Technology Screen* and the *Technology Guidelines* discussed in Section I, the education and health professional team would determine the family's technology use patterns and resulting impact areas. Based on this collated information, the child's team could determine a technology "family unplug" regime. This regime could consist of one of the following suggested technology management methods appropriate to the needs of the family, to successfully move the child and their family onto more healthy technology usage patterns: *Technology Reduction, Limited Technology Unplug*, or *Complete Technology Unplug*.

Technology Management Options

1. **Technology Reduction** consistent with expert recommendations (1-2 hours per day for children, no technology for infants) for a three month period. This option requires extensive support and weekly visits from either the education or health professional to ensure the family is able to follow through with the prescribed technology reduction protocol. As *Technology Reduction* is the least intrusive technology management method, it would likely only be useful for families with mild technology overuse problems, but not likely to prove effective in more extreme technology usage scenarios.

2. *Limited* **Technology Unplug** for two weeks, followed by technology reduction to levels within guidelines for an additional ten week period. While a more difficult intervention than the *Technology Reduction*, this method allows the family to experience life without technology, and then to use this knowledge to plan methods for the family to better manage their technology use. The *Limited Technology Unplug* method would be useful for families with significant technology overuse

problems, but who also have sufficient resources and skills to successfully manage both the technology "unplug" and the reduction periods.

3. ***Complete* Technology Unplug** for a full three months. This method obviously requires extensive support and monitoring, and should be used only in family scenarios where technology usage is extremely high and resulting behaviors are dangerous to both the child and their family. Unmanageable obesity, severe developmental delay, pervasive mental illness, uncontrolled family violence, severe learning disabilities, or evidenced parental neglect or abuse would warrant a *Complete Technology Unplug*. As this method could have adverse results similar to removal of an addictive substance, care should be given to provide extensive interventions by trained professionals to help the family acquire alternative interests and skills prior to the *Complete Technology Unplug* procedure.

These three technology management methods would be best enacted by informed and skilled education and health professionals who are trained to use a variety of supportive technology management tools and techniques.

If a child is already taking psychotropic medication for problem behavior, use of the *Technology Screen* is still indicated. If the child in question is found to use significantly higher amounts of technology than what experts recommend, then encouraging the parents to reduce technology use would be the first step. If the child's behavior subsequently improves, then possibly the child's physician may want to consider medication reduction. In *no case* should the parent ever attempt medication reduction without the guidance of the family physician, pediatrician, or psychiatrist. Without medical advice, psychotropic medication reduction could put the child at risk of harm. This potential for harm is due to the fact that psychotropic medication, when used in children, is highly toxic and addictive, especially if the child is taking multiple medications (Breggin, 2009). This toxicity can result in significant withdrawal symptoms if the medication is suddenly stopped, and therefore requires the supervision and guidance from a trained health professional

Tools for Health Professionals

TECHS-NO Rx Pad

Following use of the *Technology Screen* profiled in Section I, health professionals might consider handing out the following TECHS-NO! Rx to children who are high users of technology. This Rx is especially effective for children who have difficult and problematic behaviors, and is recommended as an alternative to behavior diagnosis and prescription of psychotropic medication. Use of the TECHS-NO! Rx is advised as a first line intervention for families of children who overuse technology. This tool can be quite effective for families when used in conjunction with the *Ten Steps to Successfully Unplug Your Child From Technology* located in Chapter 27 of *Virtual Child*. The TECHS-NO Rx pad can be ordered from the *Zone'in* website zonein.ca.

Routine Technology Screening and Intervention

NAME: _____ DATE: _____

TECHS-NO! R~x~

Technology: 1 - 2 hours per day maximum

Exercise: 3 - 4 hrs per day

Connection: listen, hugs, bedtime stories

Home: no TV's in bedrooms; no tech dinners, Sundays and holidays; no media violence

School: no tech recess and lunch

Nature: explore green space

Outdoors: play, jump, run and breathe!

SIGNATURE: _____

Need help?
www.zonein.ca   © 2009 Zone'in Programs Inc.

Chapter 32

TeleHealth or TeleDeath?

I recently received a number of questions from education and health professionals regarding the efficacy of telehealth procedures which use telecommunication systems to facilitate the delivery of child health-related information and services. A few examples are:

1. A school principal questioned whether or not telehealth was effective for speech and language services;
2. An occupational therapist questioned the efficacy of telehealth for a pediatric school-based population after she was told by her school district that she was required to use telehealth to deliver OT services to reduce her travel expenditures;
3. A speech and language pathologist who had been providing telehealth conjointly with 1:1 therapy services, stated her telehealth service "wasn't working" and she questioned whether or not she was doing it "correctly".

These questions from the education and health sectors profile just some of the concerns regarding the increased use of questionable telehealth services for treating the pediatric population, and indicate the need for additional research and information prior to escalating the use of these services with the pediatric population.

What is telehealth?

The term "telehealth" is broadly used in research literature, and can be used to reference any of the following: video conferencing between health care professionals and clients, client education or training, and may also reference client assessment, treatment intervention and follow up consultation. Related terminologies found in the literature are *ehealth, telemedicine, telerehabilitation* and *teleoccupational therapy*. This generalization of the term "telehealth" in the literature creates obvious difficultly when considering the scope of therapeutic practice. Variability in client parameters (age, diagnosis, mobility, etc.), choice of assessment and treatment type, competency level of a specific therapist, frequency/duration/intensity of intervention, and treatment environment are but a few factors to consider when regarding the efficacy of telehealth service delivery. Trying to determine cost-effectiveness and efficacy of a telehealth service requires research that is specific to each variable parameter encountered.

Who is doing telehealth?

It appears that telehealth is present to some degree in almost all health care disciplines, yet exactly what type of telehealth is offered, and whether this telehealth is actually effective, is difficult to determine when reviewing existing telehealth research. In the field of pediatrics telehealth is present in "virtually" all child care centers, hospitals, mental health clinics, private therapy clinics, and even many schools now use telehealth. As telehealth technology expands its role from video conferencing into areas of assessment and treatment, more and more health professionals are using telehealth with limited knowledge of the above noted usage parameters. Careful design of implementation protocols and preliminary review of evidence-based research is imperative prior to using telehealth on a wide scale, particularly with the pediatric population. A brief Google search indicates that a number of private practice pediatric occupational and speech and language clinics are currently offering telehealth services, yet not one of these websites cited evidence-based research outcomes, nor did they delineate telehealth service delivery protocols or procedures. Telehealth is a relatively new treatment modality, and requires careful evaluation of existing relevant research and extensive planning prior to implementation.

Does telehealth work?

The *National Initiative for Telehealth Guidelines, Environmental Scan of Organizational, Technology, Clinical and Human Resource Issues*, prepared by the NIFTE Research Consortium published April 30, 2003 is a comprehensive document on telehealth. This publication ultimately recommended that health care systems move forward to implement telehealth services, despite citing research that profiles the lack of any evidentiary base for clinical efficacy and cost-effectiveness. The publication may be helpful to readers who are seeking to design implementation protocols with outcome measures for the use of telehealth in their school or clinic settings. The following statement is excerpted from the NIFTE Executive Summary:

"The clinical efficacy and cost-effectiveness of telehealth has been demonstrated for some but not all applications. It has been asserted that technological improvements are overcoming many current limitations such that there are or soon will be no important clinical difference between face-to-face and telehealth consultations."

Telehealth Clinical Issues

The following considerations for clinical practice are excerpted from the NIFTE Executive Summary, "Clinical Issues" section.

Communication – As there is no consensus as to whether telehealth enhances or attenuates the therapeutic relationship or the traditional practice of medicine, further research is urgently needed on the nature and content of the communication process.

Standards/Quality of Clinical Care – There is diversity of opinion regarding whether there is a need for telehealth-specific practice guidelines, or if existing guidelines from the various professional licensing bodies and associations serve the purpose. The "appropriate" standard of care delivered via telehealth should be equivalent to the standard expected in traditional provision of care. If equivalent standard of care cannot be met, the telehealth practitioner needs to consider what the alternatives are and decide if it is acceptable to proceed.

Clinical Outcomes - Telehealth systems require assessment of relevant outcome data to promote and support the sustainability of telehealth programs. Telehealth networks need to have a systematic method of collecting, evaluating and reporting meaningful outcome data, which would include indicators of efficiency of service and clinical effectiveness between telehealth practitioners and patients. Telehealth should be *integrated* into the normal provision of health care services to enhance, not *replace* existing health care services and to improve access, appropriate use, and efficiency of health care services.

Telehealth Considerations

Creating a technological interface between therapist and child removes the "human element", an energetic connection that requires face to face interaction. Occupational therapists are trained in the "therapeutic use of self" which is the true gold standard for achieving effective therapy. In the absence of a therapeutic relationship, the role of the therapist is reduced to that of an observer, which, while useful, yields limited information and may significantly alter treatment recommendations. If telehealth is used for the purpose of interactive communication between therapist and child, how might children interpret the concepts of "self" and "other" when viewing their therapist through the screen? The therapist might be perceived by the child to have an appearance similar to a television character. Interacting with a real therapist vs. a virtual image could change the ways in which the child performs or verbalizes. To consider the term "self" (child or therapist) is the same concept whether using a technological interface, or face to face interaction, is denying the fact that we are all human beings whose survival and well being depends on our ability to form healthy attachments and connections with each other. Can a child actually form an attachment with a character on a screen, and can communication be therapeutic if the therapist is not perceived as real?

In pediatric occupational therapy, the use of touch, movement and human connection are three critical modalities used to facilitate child development and ensure efficacy of treatment techniques. These critical modalities are not achievable using telehealth. Relying solely on the therapist's ability to observe, and not interact, with a child will yield a poverty of information which may result in misguided treatment interventions.

Just as with teleEducation, the rapid advancement of technology into the health care system has caught professionals unaware and unprepared for the consequences of unrestricted and pervasive use of telehealth services. Thinking that telehealth will prove effective (eventually) in every setting with every individual is short sighted and will likely result in client harm. For example, proceeding forward with telerehabilitation services in school-based settings without adequate evidence-based research to support such initiatives, may increase the wait time until the client actually receives his/her research-proven 1:1 therapeutic interventions. There are inherent problems associated with the idea that technology is useful for every condition and situation, and even more inherent problems when society chooses to ignore the detrimental consequences of technology use on children. 30% of children enter school developmentally delayed and 15% have a diagnosed mental illness, both of these are associated with sedentary technology use. Yet – we are using technology to assess and provide interventions to treat these very disorders that are a *result* of technology overuse.

Restrictive use of telehealth is recommended until such time as specific research provides evidence to support implementation. Specific guidelines regarding utilization of telehealth must be developed to promote "best practice" and result in improvements (not erosions) in occupational therapy service delivery.

Government - Creating Infrastructures

The first step for governments to take to manage balanced technology use, would be to team with researchers in order to better understand the impact of technology on family, school and community structures. Because technology is evolving so rapidly, it is imperative that governments develop whole new departments to monitor each new phase of technology evolution. Based on the collated research information, the government role would be to determine child health guidelines for technology use in homes, schools and communities, and then enact management initiatives to ensure children balance participation in activities that help them grow and succeed, with technology use. While many readers would sorely disagree with government having a role in the home environment, many children are suffering abuse and neglect from parents who have technology addictions, and are therefore considered to be "at risk". Even some pre-school, daycare and school environments are placing children at risk through overuse of technology. Guidelines need to be determined, the public must be educated, regulations implemented, and legislation enacted to create safe environments in which to our raise children.

Chapter 33

Education, Regulation, Legislation

When considering impact of technology overuse by children, there are three potential roles for government to take to ensure safe use of technology by children; those roles are education, regulation and legislation. Governments could be actively involved in *educating* communities regarding inherent risks of technology use, *regulating* technology production corporations to ensure products are safe with risk warnings and *legislating* appropriate age limits and extent of violent media content.

There is a great deal of work to do in the area of government education, regulation and legislation regarding the impact of technology on children, and it goes far beyond the scope of *Virtual Child*. Following are some questions that require further investigation and consideration by government *Foundation Team* members, and could be used as a template for further planning sessions. Here are just a few questions being asked by parents, teachers, health professionals, and researchers not only in North America, but on a world stage.

Consumer Education: should governments be required to educate consumers about the possibility of product use harming our children?

Technology Screening: should government mandate routine technology screenings for children who demonstrate problems associated with high levels of technology use?

Unplug – Don't Drug: should government regulate prescriptions of psychotropic medication for problematic child behavior, by mandating prior technology "unplug" trials?

Risk Management: what is the role of governments in the area of "risk management" regarding child use of technology products?

Safe Technology: what is the role of government in regulating technology production corporations to ensure their technology is "safe" for child use?

Technology Product Research: who should do it, and should governments perform independent research regarding product safety to address potential conflict of interest?

Educational Technology: what regulatory role should government take in the area of educational technology product research regarding efficacy in the education sector?

Balanced Technology Management Initiatives for Government

Following are some *Balanced Technology Management* initiative suggestions that education, health and children and family governments can enact to chart the long path toward ensuring children balance the activities they need to grow and succeed with technology use. These immediate initiatives will assist governments in the long term development of child health guidelines to minimize the negative impact of technology on child health and academic performance.

1. Ensure all *education and health professionals* receive accurate information regarding the impact of technology on children, and are aware of *Balanced Technology Management* initiatives for six sectors.
2. Accurate and immediate up to date *consumer education* regarding inherent risks associated with technology products.
3. Helpful *consumer information* regarding effective technology management

strategies.

4. *Technology product literature* development detailing possible risks associated with use of technology product.
5. *Technology product modifications* to reduce impact on child physical, mental, social and academic health.
6. *Inclusion of Balanced Technology Management* initiatives in all government sponsored parenting courses.
7. *Community involvement initiatives* to support alternate activities, as well as sponsorship and promotion of a yearly "Unplug" week.
8. *Partnering with technology production corporations* to attain funding for initiatives that reduce the impact of technology on children e.g. school gym and playground equipment, nature access.
9. *Establish online help networks* for children who self identify a technology addiction.
10. *Add printing back into the curriculum*, and create standards for printing instruction and evaluation.
11. *Restrict the use of technology* in pre-school, daycare and elementary school settings.
12. Mandate *all education technologies pass evidenced-based criteria* for use e.g. independent, valid and reliable research studies.
13. *Regulate* the use of psychotropic medication with all children.
14. Mandate *risk warning* placement on all technology products.
15. Require *playgrounds* in school and community settings *meet minimum criteria* for achieving adequate child sensory and motor development.
16. Sponsor school and community *media literacy programs*.
17. Form *Balanced Technology Management Foundation Teams* with national, provincial, state and local organizations.

Balanced Technology Management Stamp of Approval

Government might consider offering technology production corporations a *Balanced Technology Management* (BTM) "stamp of approval" for those companies who meet designated product criteria and demonstrate they are actively working toward reversing damage caused by technology. This stamp of approval could serve as a government endorsed notification to parents, teachers and health professionals that the technology product in question meets BTM criteria of enhancing, and not eroding, child physical, mental, social and academic health.

Researchers - Keeping Up With Technology

Never before in the history of humankind has the sustainability of our species been so under the threat of destruction as it is now from the forces of technology. It falls on the shoulders of child health researchers world wide to enact immediate child health guidelines regarding child technology use. Researchers should be appointed senior advisory positions with health, education, and children and family governments to enact technology regulatory and legislative policy. The very sustainability of our children is now in question, and the time to act is now.

Cris Rowan, Author

The shear speed with which technology is evolving indicates that researchers will be required to develop new and innovative research techniques in order to track the profound ramifications on children. In the time it takes to develop a research proposal, gain funding, implement and evaluate the research, and finally publish in a respected peer reviewed journal, the research is practically antiquated. New technologies are being developed as we speak, with new platforms and programs that will change many of the applications of previous technology research. For example, the recent development of hand held devices has made it possible for children to access multiple types of technology from just about anywhere. Children can use their iPads wherever there is a wireless signal such as stores, schools, movie theatres, restaurants, and even bathrooms. Monitoring this prevalent technology use is every researcher's nightmare, requiring reliance on self reports from children, parents and teachers. Unrestricted technology use not only in the home, but also in schools, has created additional problems for child health researchers as school systems often don't participate in heath related research due to ethical restrictions.

Technology is constantly changing, and its impact on children has historically been so profound and pervasive that child physical, mental, social and academic parameters are rapidly changing as well. An example of the changing parameters is developmental milestones. In the 1980's and 90's pediatricians and therapists would educate parents that infants should be able to sit unsupported by six months of age, and stand unsupported by one year. Now, due to profound developmental delays, health professionals are reporting previous milestones, but adding "it is not unheard of" for a child to be 3-6 months delayed. This "normalization" of developmental delay by the health professional serves to appease parents, but slowly has the effect of everyone forgetting what normal development really is. Standardized tests are no longer viable ways of measuring childhood development, as testing standards created even ten years ago are far from the 21st century norm. Researchers have their work cut out for them, and will likely need to totally revamp their methods of research, design and funding, while still procuring accurate and reproducible results, in order to speed up the process to meet the pace of technology evolution.

Chapter 34

Creating Child Health Guidelines

The first step to address problems associated with technology research is for researchers to further delineate the impact technology use has on child development and academic performance. Using the *Technology Guidelines* will assist researchers in more thoroughly investigating all of the current technology usage parameters. Child age, type of technology, frequency/duration/intensity, and impact on physical, mental, social and academic factors are but a few of the routine areas that should be reflected in current research designs. Addressing all these parameters will provide rich and useful information for the eventual development of *Child Health Guidelines* for use of technology products.

The next step after completion of *Child Health Guidelines* for technology use, would be for child health researchers to team with education and health governments. Working together, researchers and government could investigate the potential risks and benefits of child technology product use *prior* to technology production and marketing. Governments working with child health researchers could mandate technology production corporations to submit products for independent research *prior* to mass production, to ensure not only product safety, but also to determine technology usage parameters.

The following considerations for child health researchers are but a few of the areas of concern that require immediate attention to ensure children engage in balance between activities they need for growth and success with technology use. Addressing these concerns will serve to assist in adult management of child balanced participation in activities that help them grow and succeed with technology use.

Risk Management: what is the role of the child health researcher in the area of risk management regarding child use of technology products, and should the risks and benefits of all child technology products be investigated by independent researchers prior to production and marketing?

Safe Technology: how much is too much? Consider the usage parameters of age, type of technology, frequency/duration/intensity, and area of impact on physical, mental, social and academic performance.

Consumer Education: is it the responsibility of researchers in conjunction with government to provide consumers *Child Health Guidelines* for technology products?

Unplug – Don't Drug: is child technology addiction misdiagnosed as a behavior disorder, and if so, what should health professionals do as a first line intervention in the treatment of child behavior disorder?

Psychotropic Medication: what are the long term implications of psychotropic medication use in children in the areas of stunted growth, poor academic performance, cardiac sudden death, aggression, suicide, and addiction?

Standardized Testing: when child development milestones are changing so rapidly, is standardized testing really a valid measure of a child's ability? Is it misleading for education and health professionals or researchers to re-standardize existing tests?

It is recommended that Researchers play a much more active role as government advisors in the area of child technology overuse, especially in the establishment of *Child Health Guidelines*. Researchers might also want to consider development of a universal and structured method of communication with media and press to ensure accurate reporting of research results along with recommendations for reversing this worrisome trend to overuse technology. Frequently media only reports the research, and fails to follow through with important information for parents, teachers and therapists regarding recommendations for managing technology use.

Balanced Technology Management Initiatives for Researchers

The following suggestions would assist child health researchers in the formation of a very long list of tasks necessary to ensure sustainable futures for our children.

1. *Child health researcher education* regarding the impact of technology use on child physical, mental, social and academic health.
2. Investigate the *impact of technology overuse* on child sensory and motor development, stress response, immune system, and cardiovascular health.
3. Determine the extent and impact of *technology addictions in children.*
4. Investigate child behavior diagnosis and technology addictions.
5. Devise safe parameters for technology use by children.
6. Uniform and structured translation of research into *consumer information* regarding general risks associated with technology products.
7. *Technology product literature* development detailing possible risks inherent in use of technology products.
8. *Technology product modification recommendations* to reduce impact on child physical, mental, social and academic health.
9. *Joint research with technology production corporations* to ensure product demonstrates minimal risk and maximal benefit for child development and academic performance.
10. Determine long term outcomes of *replacing teachers with technology.*

Technology Production Corporations – Do No Harm

Technology production corporations are like a bull in a china shop that no one knows what to do with. They have wreaked havoc in every corner of the globe, yet everyone just moves aside to welcome more. We not only ignore the devastation caused by technology production corporations, but actually seem to welcome its pervasive presence in our lives.

Cris Rowan, Pediatric Occupational Therapist and Author

How much longer will our society continue to allow technology production corporations to unconsciously destroy the very fabric with which we have created and structured our lives? Forming *Balanced Technology Management Foundation Teams* made up of parents, teachers, health professionals, government, researchers, and yes – technology production corporations, will enable us to tackle this seemingly insurmountable problem head on. Forming *Balanced Technology Management* initiatives around the premise of "Do No Harm", will enable us to start the process of reining in the technology corporations with restrictive guidelines to ensure their products don't harm our children.

Requesting that technology corporations form partnerships with schools and communities to fund child health initiatives, will further serve to bring these corporations under the regulatory "wing" of governments and child health researchers. These types of partnerships will also serve the purpose of improving the information flow between researchers and technology production corporations, and facilitate planning and implementing preliminary research prior to mass production of potentially harmful technology.

Chapter 35

Violence Reduction

When Craig Anderson and Douglas Gentile, researchers with the Iowa State University and authors of *Violent Video Game Effects on Children: Theory, Research and Public Policy*, discovered that it was the numbers of "kills" children make during video game play that was associated with consequent aggression, it seemed logical to simply reduce the frequency with which a child can induce a "kill". As my discussions with technology production corporations did not engender any support for suggested methods of reducing "kill" frequency, this may be an area that government would need to regulate. It would be interesting to find out if indeed it is the number of "kills" that children find so attractive in video games. Possibly there might be another aspect to video games other than killing that will still appeal to the general public, but not elicit so much child aggression.

It is highly unlikely that technology production corporations (without government regulatory control) would be willing to modify their products, if the end result would be reduced sales. Survey research could determine the minimum number of "kills" per minute that would be required to satisfy the masses, and then this could be the regulated limit. For example, numbers of "kills" could be regulated to a maximum of 10 "kills" per minute, which could be limited by bullet or weapon restrictions. While the child is waiting, they could be buying more ammunition or supplies, or pass some sort of test to acquire more weaponry. I'm sure the video game designers could come up with some interesting alternatives to mass killing.

One of the options I offered to technology production corporations for reducing media violence was to educate video game designers on the aspects of child health that are negatively affected by technology overuse. Just as parents are uninformed in this area, so are producers of violent media content. I'm not saying that everyone once informed will convert to less violent content, but possibly they might be motivated toward exploring alternative options. Possibly increasing the shooter difficulty, by making the shooter a sniper, or someone who needs to hide and can only shoot when opportunity permits, would be an option. The targets could be harder to get a clear shot at because the target or the shooter would be constantly moving, because they are driving a car, or are on a moving object such as a boat or plane. Maybe the shooter should bury his/her dead, which would occupy time spent on an activity alternate to killing. More obstacles in the shooter's path, or more complicated plots would also slow down the kills. Players might have to shoot a few people, but they would also have to perform lock picking, spying or gathering information about their opponent's whereabouts as well. Other alternatives are instead of focusing on killing others, video games could be redesigned to sublimate aggression, sort of like an interactive version of "capture the flag".

Media violence in movies and television shows has escalated to the point where it does not seem remotely possible to pack in any more "kills", even if the producers wanted to. The action is moving so fast and furious in movies that the plot is rarely discernable, if there even is a plot. I asked a CBC film producer why the pace is so fast that the viewer can't even follow the plot, and he told me that it is the *production companies* that force this type of film production. I thought it was sort of odd that no one consults the viewer as to what type of production they would like. Who likes the script being scrolled at the bottom of the newscast? Or who likes the next show being constantly advertised at the bottom of the current show's screen? No one has asked me these questions!

It doesn't seem like video game designers or television producers want to be educated on their contribution to our children's overuse of technology. I was recently informed by a colleague who had attended a video game convention that the big push now is for non-technology related product manufacturers to sell "tokens" for video games. When specific products get shown on television commercials, the product manufacturer would monitor viewer attention through use of an eye-tracing camera on top of their television. If the viewer's eyes are attentive on the screen during the full commercial, the viewer gets to download tokens for their favorite video game. As invasive as token economy sounds, this type of marketing is coming into living rooms faster and faster. What happens when someone hacks into this system, and starts watching viewers, or records them and posts their every action and words on Facebook for everyone to see?

We are rapidly moving into a perilous time regarding the ramifications of unchecked technology production, specifically the production of violent video games.

Chapter 36

Product Harm and Risk Warnings

Technology production corporations would be advised to work in conjunction with government and child health researchers to enact sufficient changes to technology products to ensure sustainable futures for all children. The first step toward responsibility for "product harm" would be for technology production corporations to understand the impact of inevitable misuse of their products, especially by children who stand the chance of sustaining long term effects. Children who would be most vulnerable to product harm would be those who have already sustained damage from overuse such as developmental delay, obesity, aggression, social and communication disorders, mental illness, poor academic performance, and learning and/or attention problems (to name a few).

The next step for technology production corporations would be to enact their own management initiatives to ensure children balance participation in activities that help them grow and succeed with technology use. Responsible use of technology requires adequate consumer risk education. Technology production corporations might want to start this process of *risk education*, prior to government regulation.

A few additional considerations for *Balanced Technology Management Foundation Team* members to discuss are listed below.

Safe Technology: should technology production corporations be required to ensure their technology is "safe" for child use; if so, how?

Consumer Education: should technology production corporations be required to educate consumers regarding possible harm from product use?

Negligence: should technology production corporations be held legally responsible, if they have neglected to inform the consumers of harmful effects from product use?

Due Diligence: what type of consumer education would be sufficient to achieve "due diligence" necessary to release technology production corporations from legal responsibility?

Risk Management: what is the role of technology production corporations in the area of risk management?

Balanced Technology Management Initiatives for Technology Production Corporations

Technology production corporations could participate in a variety of initiatives that would work toward improving child health and productivity. Providing an online "help" network for children with technology addictions is a first step toward gaining some assistance for these children. Funding of *nature* and *movement* based initiatives in schools and communities will serve to counteract some of the more sedentary aspects of technology use. Funding school nature outings such as a weekly trip to the local park, or a yearly school camping adventure, will provide attention restoration needed for optimizing productivity and academic success. Funding of school solariums or conservatory additions for creation of attention restorative "green space", would serve to counteract the negative effects of technology on learning. Providing monetary support for community programs that promote family activities would serve to detach family members from technology and reattach them to each other, suck as sponsoring free recreation center passes during a community technology "unplug" week.

The following suggestions are but a few of the possible initiatives that could be enacted by technology production corporations to demonstrate responsibility for child health and success.

1. *Product information literature* should be provided with all technology products detailing risk for harmful effects on children.
2. *Consumer information* regarding managing balance between healthy activity and technology.
3. *Product modifications* enacted to enhance and not erode child physical, mental, social and academic health and performance.
4. *Media violence reduced* with reward and strategy themes for video games, and through more complex and creative plot lines for movies and television.
5. *Community involvement initiatives* to support alternate healthy activities should be formed in conjunction with schools and communities.
6. *Online help networks* for children with technology addictions, providing local resource information for counseling and self help programs. A "blog" would be helpful to assist children in feeling as if they are not alone.

Balanced Technology Management Health Approved Status

Participating technology production corporations could receive the *Balanced Technology Management* (BTM) "stamp of approval" from government regulatory bodies, which notifies parents, teachers and health professionals that their product meets BTM criteria of enhancing child physical, mental, social and academic health.

Conclusion – Are Virtual Children Sustainable?

It's not about the next generation of technology, it's about the next generation of human beings. We may discover very soon that technology and human survival are mutually exclusive.

Cris Rowan, Occupational Therapist, Speaker and Author

If the evolution of society is measured by how well it takes care of its most vulnerable, in this case – children, then North American society fails miserably. The "de-evolution" of society would be a good way to describe trends reported in *Virtual Child*. Over the course of the past 50,000 years, humans have managed to rise to the top of the food chain to dominate all other life forms on planet earth. Until quite recently (in the last 50 years), humans have successfully functioned as "pack" animals, with each member of the group serving a vital purpose and role. Darwin's "survival of the fittest" theory reigned true, as evolutionary stressors of disease, climate change, and predation made sure that *only the strong survive!* Movement, touch and human connection, which have always been considered to be three essential, critical factors for human species survival, were plentiful and abundant. The more physically fit human could run faster, had sharper sensory acuity for hunting and gathering, and had sufficient endurance for hard work and harsh climate conditions.

Babies, toddlers and young children spent every moment in the arms of a parent, grandparent or sibling, receiving adequate touch to enable a calm and secure individual. This continuous tactile sensory input optimized the child's development of their motor skills, which enabled them to perform a variety of required fine and gross motor tasks. Meals were spent in conversation connecting with family or friends, often in large groups, playing games or making music and dancing. Families and communities living as a "pack" not only ensured pack survival, but also offered each member ample opportunity to reach the limits of their own human potential by pushing them (often quite harshly) to succeed. If the pack member didn't rise to the occasion, and adapt to the stresses placed on them, they didn't survive. Since Darwin's time, we have known that evolution of the human species requires *adaptation* to stress, and stress serves to promote species adaptation, but only to a degree. If the stress becomes too great, the human species will cease to adapt or evolve, and extinction becomes inevitable.

In my book *Virtual Child – The Terrifying Truth About What Technology Is Doing to Children,* I have detailed recent changes to human biology resulting from technology overuse. I will now propose that humans are not adapting to these changes fast enough, or sufficient enough, to sustain human existence on this planet. For many children, the boundaries between the virtual world and the real world have started to blur, and the human body, mind and soul are becoming lost in a void which is *devoid* of movement, touch, and human connection. The rapid pace with which technology has invaded the human species has raised a host of questions, and due to the fact that present day research simply can't keep up, many of these questions have no answers. For example, what intensity, frequency and duration of evolutionary stress, in the form of technology, can the human species realistically adapt to? As rapidly as technology is advancing, can human species adaptation possibly keep up, and what happens if it can't? These questions are posed to the reader as food for further thought, and action. Technology is a "train" that has moved out of the station and is rapidly accelerating. Humans are starting to fall off the *technology train* at an incrementally increasing rate, often without the knowledge or awareness of the closest members of their pack, their families, educators and health professionals. Children, who are truly the most vulnerable members of any pack or society, appear to be falling off the *technology train* the fastest, in increasing record numbers, and are therefore fairing the worst. Bringing the *technology train* back to the station will provide adequate time to understand the impact of technology on child health and academic performance. With mounting research showing technology is harming children, it is time to take immediate measures to restrict technology use, and begin to manage a *balance* between what children need to grow and succeed, with technology.

Evolution and Child Sustainability

Sustainability is defined by the Wikapedia dictionary as the capacity to *endure*. Wikapedia goes on to state that from an ecological perspective, the term sustainability describes how biological systems remain *productive* over time. For humans, sustainability is defined as the potential for long-term maintenance of *well being*.

Delving further into the question of whether today's children of technology are sustainable for generations to come, I will proceed to discuss the effects of technology overuse on children's physical, mental, social and academic performance, with reference made to these three definitions of sustainability – *endurance, productivity*, and *well being*. While some readers might find this notion to be quite esoteric and far fetched, speaking as a biologist with an interest in promoting sustainable environments, this is an area that I am hoping will peak interest and debate. If the way in which society is using technology to raise and educate children is indeed not sustainable as I propose, then we as a society owe it to future generations of children to change our ways. There is a lot of work to be done, and quickly, if we are to turn the tide and start taming the powerful force that technology is exerting on our lives. Each and every one of us would be wise to ask of ourselves "Who is driving the ship? Technology – or me?"

Delayed child development associated with overuse of technology, is unlikely to cause *species demise* in and of itself. However, when considering the secondary effects of delayed development on family socioeconomic status and academic performance, species demise could become a reality. Suboptimal sensory and motor development in children impacts on their achievement of literacy, which in turn impacts on a child's completion of high school. Failure to complete high school affects job acquisition and future potential as a wage earner, to say nothing of the economic impact of high school "drop-outs" on the community as a whole. Failure to complete high school also affects attractiveness for human mating and formation of eventual partnerships, affecting overall species *productivity* and *endurance*.

Obesity secondary to technology overuse is associated with diabetes and cardiovascular disorders, both affecting species *endurance* and *well being*. Child mental health impairment, associated with technology overuse, impacts on species *productivity* and *well being*. Poor communication skills and social isolation, both traits causally related to technology overuse in children, have a negative impact on species prowess and ability to find a mate. Unsuitability for mating will limit human ability to form meaningful relationships necessary to form partnerships and raise a family. Inability to secure a life partner and raise a family affects species propagation, and hence affects overall human sustainability through impacting *endurance* and *well being*. Rising use of psychotropic medication with young children to treat behavior disorders associated with technology overuse has the potential to negatively impact all three sustainability factors - *endurance, productivity*, and *well being*. While child aggression may have been advantageous to species longevity 100 years ago, in the 21st century child aggression is now coupled with developmental delay, impulsivity and illiteracy, making this trait far less attractive when considering overall species sustainability.

The ability of a child to adapt to sensory responses in their environment emerges early in life as a protective and discriminative mechanism, and as children grow they typically become better at tolerating uncomfortable sensory stimuli by applying strategies to self regulate (Dunn, 2007). Sensory over-responsivity reflects a failure to achieve a balance between sensitization and habituation, and can affect many aspects of a child's ability to function in both home and school settings (Ben-Sasson, 2010). The impact of technology overuse on a developing child's sensory system, and that sensory system's ability to adapt and habituate to technological stimuli is unknown at this time. Possibly the profound rise in child mental and behavioral disorders reflects the fact that children are not adapting to the chaotic and hyper stimulated world of technology as well as we might think.

The ability to relate in meaningful ways with other human beings, to be able to empathize and sympathize with others, really sets the human species distinctly apart from the animal species. As empathy requires human relatedness, one might ask the question "What will be the end result of technology's progression toward isolation of the human species?" Sedentary, detached, angry, obese, over-stimulated and isolated, how much longer can the new millennium child attempt to adapt to this unhealthy lifestyle, and at what point is the human species no longer sustainable?

The physical and mental status of the parent is also a crucial factor for determining how well the child will fare. Parent obesity, mental illness, addictions, social isolation, and aggression, all conditions associated with technology overuse, have the potential to have profound effects on the *endurance, productivity,* and *well being* of the next generation. Long durations of attachment to technology effectively "detaches" parents from their children, not only impacting on the parent's ability to provide sustenance such as food, shelter and clothing, but also negatively impacting on the life sustaining effects of healthy attachment formation between parent and child.

In conclusion, evidence suggests that parents and schools allow young children extended periods of unrestricted access to various forms of technology which is harmful to their physical, mental, social and academic development. Further evidence suggests parents are increasingly presenting their children to physicians for assessment of complex behavior disorders that may be linked to the physical inactivity and sensory over-responsivity inherent in the overuse of technology, or related to the "detached" state of the parent.

Health and education professional routine monitoring of technology use through application of a *Technology Screen* would be a start toward achieving eventual *Balanced Technology Management*, and consequently serve to improve the health and academic performance of children. Implementation of the school-based *Creating Sustainable Futures Program*, and formation of community-based *Balanced Technology Management Foundation Teams*, would ensure species sustainability. Children with high technology usage may benefit from a technology "unplug" trial of one to three months prior to costly behavior diagnosis and potentially harmful prescription of psychotropic medication. Educators may consider implementation of school-based media literacy programs, which have proven effective in reducing technology use and obesity (Robinson, 1999). Recommendations for family disconnection from technology and reconnection with each other and nature, would go a long way toward reversing these worrisome societal trends.

Research References

Active Healthy Kids Canada [2008 report card on the internet]. Available from: http://www.activehealthykids.ca/Ophea/ActiveHealthyKids_v2/upload/AHKC-Short-Form-EN.pdf.

Anderson CA, Berkowitz, L, Donnerstein E, Huesmann LR, Johnson JD, Linz D, Malamuth NM, Wartella E. The Influence of Media Violence on Youth. *Psychological Science in the Public Interest.* 2003; 4:81-110.

Anderson C. A., Gentile D. A. & Buckley, K. E. *Violent Video Game effects on Children and Adolescents: Theory, Research and Public Policy.* Oxford University Press; Oxford, UK. 2007.

Autism Society of Canada. (2010). Retrieved April 30, 2010, from http://www.autismsocietycanada.ca/asd_research/research_prevalence/index_e.html

Autism Society. (2010). Retrieved April 30, 2010, from http://www.autism-society.org/site/Clubs?club_id=1217&sid=9320&pg=news

Ayres JA. Sensory integration and learning disorders. California: Western Psychological Services; 1972.

Baranek, G. T., David, F. J., Poe, M. D., Stone, W. L. & Watson, L. R. Sensory Experiences Questionnaire: discriminating sensory features in young children with autism, developmental delays, and typical development. *Journal of Child Psychology and Psychiatry.* 2006;47(6):591–601.

Baron-Cohen S. Atypical sensory functioning in autism spectrum conditions. Research in progress at Autism Research Center, Cambridge, UK. http://www.autismresearchcentre.com/research/project.asp?id=3

Barros RM, Silver EJ, Stein RE. School Recess ad Group Classroom Behavior. *Pediatrics.* 2009; 123(2):431-436.

Bass, A. Side Effects: A Prosecutor, a Whistleblower, and the Truth About a Best Selling Antidepressant. New York: Algonquin Books, Workman Publishing Company; 2008.

Baughman F. There is No Such Thing as a Psychiatric Disorder/Disease/Chemical Imbalance. Public Library of Science Medicine. 2006; 3(7): e318. Available at: http://www.plosmedicine.org/article/info%3Adoi%2F10.1371%2Fjournal.pmed.0030318.

BBC News. Computer Game Teenager Gets DVT. January 29, 2004. Retrieved August 9, 2010 from: http://news.bbc.co.uk/2/hi/health/3441237.stm

BBC News. Obesity's huge challenge for humans. September 9, 2002. By Jonathan Amos. Available at: http://news.bbc.co.uk/2/hi/in_depth/sci_tech/2002/leicester_2002/2246450.stm

Ben-Sasson, A., Carter, A. S. & Briggs-Gowan, M. The Development of Sensory Over-Responsivity From Infancy to Elementary School. *Journal of Abnormal Child Psychology.* (2010). DOI 10.1007/s10802-010-9435-9.

Bigelow, A. (2006). Effects of Skin-to-Skin Contact on Early Mother-Infant Interaction: Preliminary Findings from a Canadian Sample of Full-Term Infants. Paper presented at the Sixth Biennial International Workshop of the International Network of Kangaroo Mother Care in Cleveland, Ohio, October 2006. Available at: www.preciousimagecreations.com/files/still_face_studies.doc

Birmingham CL, Muller JL, Palepu A, Spinelli JJ, Anis AH. The cost of obesity in Canada. *Canadian Medical Association Journal.* 1999; 160:483-488.

Block, JJ. Issues for DSM – V: Internet Addiction. *Journal of Clinical Psychiatry.* 2008; 67 (5): 821-826.

Blumenfeld SL. Can Dyslexia be artificially induced in school? Yes, says researcher Edward Miller.http://donpotter.net/PDF/Miller-Blumenfeld_Dyslexia_Article.pdf.

Bowlby, J. *A Secure Base: Parent-Child Attachment and Healthy Human Development.* Basic Books; New York. 1990.

Boyle C.A., Decoufle' P. & Yeargin-Alsopp M. Prevalence and health impact of developmental disabilities in US children. *Pediatrics.* 1994; 93 (3): 399-403.

Braswell J, Rine R. Evidence that vestibular hypofunction affects reading acuity in children. *International Journal of Pediatric Otorhinolaryngology.* 2006; 70 (11): 1957-1965.

Breggin, P. *Medication Madness: The Role of Psychiatric Drugs in Cases of Violence, Suicide and Murder.* St. Martin's Press; New York, NY. 2008.

Bristol University: School for Policy Studies News (October 11, 2010). *Screen time linked to psychological problems in children.* Available at: http://www.bristol.ac.uk/sps/news/2010/107.html

Buchanan AM, Gentile DA, Nelson DA, Walsh DA, Hensel J. *What goes in must come out: Children's Media Violence Consumption at Home and Aggressive Behaviours at School.* Paper presented at the International Society for the Study of Behavioural Development Conference, Ottawa, Ontario, Canada. Available online at: www.mediafamily.org/research/report_issbd_2002.shtml.

Burdette, HL, Whitaker RC. A national study of neighborhood safety, outdoor play, television viewing, and obesity in preschool children. *Pediatrics.* 2005; 116: 657-662.

Canadian Standards Association - Children's Playspaces and Equipment Standard, 4th Edition. (2007). Available at: http://www.csa.ca/cm/ca/en/search/article/childrens-playspaces-and-equipment-standard-fourth-edition

CBC News. *France pulls plug on TV shows aimed at babies* [CBC online article Wednesday, August 20, 2008]. Available from: http://www.cbc.ca/world/story/2008/08/20/french-baby.html.

CBC News. ADHD Drug Linked to Suicide Attempts: Health Canada. CBC News July 3,

2008. Available at: http://www.cbc.ca/health/story/2008/07/03/adhd-drug-warning.html.

CBS News. Mar 13, 2008, Man Sentenced For Killing Toddler Over Broken Xbox. Available at: http://cbs3.com/local/Tyrone.Spellman.Xbox.2.676702.html

CBC News. August 16, 2010. Ontario School Board won't turn off Wi-Fi. Available at: http://www.cbc.ca/canada/windsor/story/2010/08/16/wifi-students.html

Center for Disease Control and Prevention – Diabetes Public Health Resource. (2010). Available at: http://www.cdc.gov/diabetes/projects/cda2.htm

Centre for Disease Control and Prevention. 2003. Mental Health in the United States: Prevalence of Diagnosis and Medication Treatment for Attention Deficit/Hyperactivity Disorder. Available from: www.cdc.gov/mmwr/preview/mmwrhtml/mm5434a2.htm.

Center on Media and Child Health, Boston Children's Hospital. Available at: www.cmch.tv

Children, adolescents and television. American Academy of Pediatrics, Committee on Public Education. Pediatrics. 2001; 107 (2): 423-426.

Children, adolescents and advertising. Committee on Communications, American Academy of Pediatrics. Pediatrics. 2006; 118 (6): 2562-2569.

Christakis, D. A., Gilkerson, J., Richards, J. A., Zimmerman, F. J., Garrison, M. M., Xu, D., Gray, S. & Yapanel, U. Audible Television and Decreased Adult Words, Infant Vocalizations, and Conversational Turns. *Archives of Pediatrics & Adolescent Medicine.* 2009;163(6):554-558. Available at: http://archpedi.amaassn.org/cgi/content/full/163/6/554#AUTHINFO

Christakis DA, Zimmerman FJ. Violent Television During Preschool Is Associated With Antisocial Behavior During School Age. *Pediatrics.* 2007; 120: 993-999.

Christakis DA, Zimmerman FJ, DiGiuseppe DL, McCarty CA. Early television exposure and subsequent attentional problems in children. *Pediatrics.* 2004; 113 (4): 708-713.

Committee on Public Education. Media Violence. 2001; 108:1222-1226. Available at: http://www.mediafamily.org/videogame2006summit/publications.shtml.

Crane, L., Goddard, L. & Pring, P. Sensory processing in adults with autism spectrum disorders. *Autism.* 2009; 13, 215-228.

Crittenden, P. M.. Raising Parents: Attachment, Parenting and Child Safety. Willan Publishing; Oxfordshire, UK. 2008.

Davidson, K. & Bressler, S. Piloting a points-based caseload measure for community based paediatric occupational and physiotherapists. *Canadian Journal of Occupational Therapy.* 2010;77(3):174-180.

Diagnosis and Statistical Manual, Fifth Edition. Available at www.DSMV.org.

DeBerardis D, D'Albenzio A, Gambi F, Sepede G, Valchera A, Conti CM, Fulcheri M, Cavuto M, Ortolani C, Salerno RM, Serroni N, Ferro FM. Alexithymia and Its Relationships with Dissociative Experiences and Internet Addiction in a Nonclinical

Sample. *CyberPsychology & Behavior*. 2008; doi:10.1089/cpb.2008.0108.

de Waal, F.. *Our Inner Ape: A Leading Primatologist Explains Why We Are Who We Are.* Riverhead Books, NY. 2005.

Diller L. H. *Running on Ritalin: A Physician Reflects on Children, Society, and Performance of a Pill.* Bantam Books; NY. 1999.

dosReis, S., Zito, J.M., Safer, D..J., Gardner, J.F., Puccia, K. B. & Owens, P.L. Multiple psychotropic medication use for youths: A two-state comparison. *Journal of Child and Adolescent Psychopharmacology*. 2005;15(1): 68-77.

Faber Taylor, A., Kuo, F. E. & Sullivan, W. C. Coping With ADD – The Surprising Connection to Green Play Settings. *Journal of Environment and Behavior.* 2001; 33(1):54-77.

Fast Company Magazine. (April, 2010). *"A" is for App*. By Anya Kamenetz. http://www.fastcompany.com/magazine/144.

Feldman, R., Eidelman, A. I., Sirota, L. & Weller, A. Comparison of Skin-to-Skin (Kangaroo) and Traditional Care: Parenting Outcomes and Preterm Infant Development. *Pediatrics.* 2002;110(1):16-26.

Field, T., Lasko, D., Mundy, P., Henteleff, T., Kabat, S., Talpins, S. & Dowling, M. Brief report: Autistic children's attentiveness and responsivity improve after touch therapy. *Journal of Autism and Developmental Disorder.* 1997: 27(3):333-338.

Flores, P. *Addiction as an Attachment Disorder.* Rowman & Littlefield Publishers Inc.; Oxford, UK. 2004.

Gangwisch, J. E., Babiss, L. A., Malaspina, D., Turner J. B., Zammit, G. K. & Posner, K. (2010). Earlier Parental Set Bedtimes as a Protective Factor Against Depression and Suicidal Ideation. *Sleep.* 33(1):96-106.

Guardian News. August 26, 2010. *Parents are forgetting how to play with their children, study shows.* Available at: http://uk.lifestyle.yahoo.com/family-parenting/parents-forgetting-play-children-study-shows-article-huib.html

Gaskin, C. J., Elsom, S. J. & Happell, B. Interventions for reducing the use of seclusion in psychiatric facilities. *British Journal of Psychiatry.* 2007;191:298-303. DOI:10.1192/bjp.bp.106.834538

Gentile D. Pathological Video-Game Use Among Youth Ages 8 to 18. *Journal of Psychological Science.* 2009; 3(2):1-9.

Gentzler, A. L., Oberhauser, A. M., Westerman, D. and Nadorff, D. K. College Students' Use of Electronic Communication with Parents: Links to Loneliness, Attachment, and Relationship Quality *Cyberpsychology, Behavior, and Social Networking.* 2010;doi:10.1089/cyber.2009.0409.

Ghassemzadeh L, Shahraray M, Moradi A. Prevalence of Internet Addiction and Comparison of Internet Addicts and Non-Addicts in Iranian High Schools. *CyberPsychology & Behavior.* 2008: doi:10.1089/cpb.2007.0243.

Globe and Mail. (2010). By Zosia Bielski. *Today's college kids are 40-per-cent less empathetic, study finds.* June 1, 1010. Available at: http://www.theglobeandmail.com/life/work/todays-college-kids-are-40-per-cent-less-empathetic-study-finds/article1587609/

Globe and Mail. (2008). By Sarah Boesveld. Virtual games, real addiction. October 22, 2008. http://www.theglobeandmail.com/life/article717627.ece

Goldberg, E. & Simner, M. A. Comparison of Children's Handwriting Under Traditional vs. Whole Language Instruction. *Canadian Journal of School Psychology.* 1999; 14(2): 11-30.

Goodwin, R., Gould, M. S., Blanco, C. & Olfson, M. Prescription of psychotropic medications to youth in office-based practices. *Psychiatric Services.* 2001; 52(8):1081-1087.

Government of Canada; *The well-being of Canada's young children* [report on the internet]. 2003. Cat. No.: RH64-20/2003, ISBN: 0-662-67443-X. Available from: http://www.socialunion.gc.ca/ecd/2003/RH64-20-2003E.pdf.

Graham, S., Harris, K., Mason, L., Fink-Chorzempa, B., Moran , S. & Saddler, B. How Do Primary Grade Teachers Teach Handwriting? A National Survey. *Reading and Writing: An Interdisciplinary Journal.* 2008: 21;49-69.

Graham, S. & Weintraub, N. A Review of Handwriting Research: Progress and Prospects from 1980 to 1994. *Educational Psychology Review.* 1996; 8, 7-87.

Graham, S., Harris, K. & Fink, B. Is Handwriting Causally Related to Learning to Write? Treatment of Handwriting Problems in Beginning Writers. *Journal of Educational Psychology.* 2000;92: 620-633.

Graham, S. *Handbook of Writing Research, Ch 13 – Strategy Instruction and the Teaching of Writing.* Guilford Press, New York. 2006.

Graham, S., MacArthur, C. & Fitzgerald, J. *Best Practices in Writing Instruction.* Guilford Press, New York. 2007.

Grandin, T. & Johnson, C. *Animals in Translation: Using the Mysteries of Autism to Decode Animal Behavior.* Simon and Schuster, New York. 2005.

Hamilton, S. Screening for developmental delay: Reliable, easy-to-use tools. *Journal of Family Practice.* 2006; 55 (5): 416-422.

Hancox, R. J., Milne, B.J. & Poulton, R. Association of television during childhood with poor educational achievement. *Archives of Pediatric and Adolescent Medicine.* 2005; 159 (7): 614-618.

Harvey-Berino, J. & Rourke, J. Obesity Prevention in Preschool Native-American Children: A Pilot Study Using Home Visiting. *Obesity Research.* 2001; 11:606-611.

Healy, J. M. *Different Learners: Identifying, Preventing, and Treating You Child's Learning Problems.* Simon and Schuster, NY. 2010.

Horvath, C. W. Measuring television addiction. *Journal of Broadcasting and Electronic*

Media. 2004; 48 (3): 378-398.

Howard, A.W. Keeping children safe: rethinking how we design our environments. *Canadian Medical Association Journal.* 2010; 182(6); 573-577.

Howard, A.W., MacArthur, C.. Willan, A, et al. The effect of safer play equipment on playground injury rates among school children. *Canadian Medical Association Journal.* 2005: 172; 1443-1446.

Huesmann, L.R. The Impact of Electronic Media Violence: Scientific Theory and Research. *Journal of Adolescent Health.* 2007; 41: S6-13.

Insel. T,R, & Young, L.J. The neurobiology of attachment. *Nature Reviews Neuroscience.* 2001; 2: 129-136.

Irwin, M. Proceedings presented at the 2009 International Center for the Study of Psychiatry and Psychology. New York.

Jennings, J.T. Conveying the message about optimal infant positions. *Physical and Occupational Therapy in Pediatrics.* 2005; 25 (3); 3-18.

Jensen, P.S. & Cooper, J.R. *Attention Deficit Hyperactivity Disorder: State of Science – Best Practices.* 2002. Chapter 10. Public Health and Toxicological Issues Concerning Stimulant Treatment for ADHD.

Joseph, J. *The Gene Illusion: Genetic Research in Psychiatry and Psychology Under the Microscope.* PCCS Books Publishing, Herefordshire, UK. 2003.

Kaiser Foundation Report. 2010. Retrieved on April 30, 2010 from http://www.kff.org/entmedia/upload/8010.pdf.

Kaplan S. The restorative benefits of nature: Toward an integrative framework. *Journal of Environmental Psychology.* 1995; 15: 169-182.

Kasteleijn-Nolst Trenite, D. G., Martins da Silva, A. & Ricci, S. Video Games are Exciting: A European Study of Video Game-Induced Seizures and Epilepsy. *Epileptic Disorders.* 2003;4; 121-128.

Kershaw, P. British Columbia Business Council and University of British Columbia researchers with the Human Early Learning Partnership. A Comprehensive Policy Framework for Early Human Capital Investment in BC. 2009. Retrieved on April 30, 2010 from www.earlylearning.ubc.ca/documents/2009/15by15-Executive-Summary.pdf.

Kessler, R.C., Adler, L., Barkley, R., Biederman, J., Conners, C. K., Demler, O,, Faraone, S. V., Greenhill, L. L., Howes, M. J., Secnik, K., Spencer, T., Ustun, T. B., Walters, E ,E. & Zaslavsky, A. M. The Prevalence and Correlates of Adult ADHD in the United States: Results for the National Comorbidity Survey Replication. *American Journal of Psychiatry.* 2006; 163:716-723.

Kirsch, I. & Antonuccio, D. FDA testimony on the efficacy of antidepressants with children. February 2004. Available from:http://www.ahrp.org/risks/SSRI0204/KirschAntonuccio.php.

Korkman. M. Introduction to the special issue on normal neuropsychological development in the school-age years. *Developmental Neuropsychology.* 2001; 20 (1):325-330.

Kowalski, R. M. & Limber, S. P. Electronic Bullying Among Middle School Students. *Journal of Adolescent Health.* 2007; 41:S22-30.

Kuo, F. E. & Faber Taylor, A. A Potential Natural Treatment for Attention-Deficit/Hyperactivity Disorder: Evidence from a National Study. *American Journal of Public Health.* 2004; 94(9):1580-1586.

Lane, S. J., Reynolds, S. & Thacker L.. Sensory over-responsivity and ADHD: differentiating using electrodermal responses, cortisol, and anxiety. *Frontiers in Integrative Neuroscience.* 2010;4 (8), 1-11. doi: 10.3389/fnint.2010.00008.

Lang, R., Koegel, L. K., Ashbaugh, K., Regester, K., Ence, W. & Smith, W. (2010). Physical exercise and individuals with autism spectrum disorders: A systematic review. Research in Autism Spectrum Disorders. DOI:10.1016/j.rasd.2010.01.006

Louv, R. *Last child in the woods: Saving our children from Nature-Deficit Disorder.* Algonquin Books; NY. 2005.

MacArthur, C., Hu, X. & Wesson, D. E. Risk factors for severe injuries associated with falls from playground equipment. *Accident Analysis and Prevention Journal.* 2000: 32(3); 377-382.

McEwan, K., Waddell, C. & Barker, J.. Bringing Children's Mental Health "Out of the Shadows". *Canadian Medical Association Journal.* 2007; 176(4): 471-472.

Mandell , D. S., Morales, K. H., Marcus, S. C., Stahmer, A. C., Doshi, J. & Polsky, D. E. Psychotropic medication use among medicaid-enrolled children with Autism Spectrum Disorders. *Pediatrics.* 2008; 121 (3): 441-449.

Mangen, A. Hypertext fiction reading: haptics and immersion. *Journal of Research.* 2008;31(4):404-419.

Mate', G. *Scattered Minds: A New Look at the Origins and the Healing of Attention Deficit Disorder.* Vintage Canada. 2000.

May-Benson, T. A., & Cermak, S. A. Development of an assessment for ideational praxis. *American Journal of Occupational Therapy.* 2007;61:148–153.

Mental Health: A Report of the Surgeon General, Overview of Mental Disorders in Children [report on the internet]. Available from: http://www.surgeongeneral.gov/library/mentalhealth/chapter2/sec2_1.html.

Merrow, J. *Below C Level: How American Education Encourages Mediocrity and What We Can Do about It.* Kindle Edition. 2010.

Montagu, A. Touching: *the Human Significance of the Skin 2nd Edition.* Harper and Row; NY. 1972.

Mukaddes, N. M., Bilge, S., Alyanak, B. & Kora, M.E. Clinical characteristics and treatment responses in cases diagnosed as Reactive Attachment Disorder. *Child Psychiatry and Human Development*. 2000; 30 (4): 273-287.

Muralidharan, S. & Fenton, M. *Containment strategies for people with serious mental illness* (Review). The Cochrane Collaboration, published in *The Cochrane Library*, Issue 4. John Wiley and Sons, Ltd. 2009.

Murray, J., Liotti, M., Ingmundson, P., Mayberg, H., Pu, Y., Zamarripa, F., Liu, Y., Woldorff, M., Gao, J. & Fox, P. Children's brain activations while viewing televised violence revealed by fMRI. *Media Psychology*. 2006; 8 (1): 25-37.

National Association for Sport and Physical Education. NASPE Releases First Ever Physical Activity Guidelines for Infants and Toddlers. February 6, 2002. Available at: http://www.aahperd.org/naspe/template.cfm?template=toddlers.html.

National Center for Education Statistics (2010). United States Department of Education: Institute of Education Sciences. Available at: http://nces.ed.gov/pubsearch/pubsinfo.asp?pubid=2000071

National Initiative for Telehealth Guidelines. *Environmental Scan of Organizational, Technology, Clinical and Human Resource Issues.* Prepared by the NIFTE Research Consortium published April 30, 2003National Center for Education Statistics, 2005. Available at: http://nces.ed.gov/.

National Institute of Mental Health. Press Release, December 14, 2009. National Survey Tracks Rates of Common Mental Disorders Among American Youth. Available at: http://www.nimh.nih.gov/science-news/2009/national-survey-tracks-rates-of-common-mental-disorders-among-american-youth.shtml

National Post. Monday, Aug. 16, 2010. *School board rejects concern Wi-Fi makes kids sick.* By Linda Nguyen. Available at: http://www.nationalpost.com/news/School+board+rejects+concern+makes+kids+sick/3404752/story.html

Nelson, M. C., Neumark-Sztainer, D.R., Hannan, P. J., Sirard, J. R. & Story, M. Longitudinal and secular trends in physical activity and sedentary behavior during adolescence. *Pediatrics*. 2006; 118 (6): 1627-1634.

News.com.au. Ohio teenager Daniel Petric killed mother over Halo 3 video game. By staff writers on January 13, 2009. Available at: http://www.news.com.au/technology/teen-killed-mother-over-video-game/story-e6frfro0-1111118553464

New York Magazine. Snooze or Loose. By Po Bronson Published Oct 7, 2007. Available at: http://nymag.com/news/features/38951/
New York Times. Researchers Fail to Reveal Full Drug Pay. The New York Times June 8, 2008. Available at: http://www.nytimes.com/2008/06/08/us/08conflict.html.

New York Times. No Einstein in Your Crib? Get a Refund. The New York Times October 23, 2009. Available at: http://www.nytimes.com/2009/10/24/education/24baby.html?_r=1.

Nielsen Quarterly Report. http://it.nielsen.com/site/documents/A2M2_3Screens_1Q09_FINAL.pdf

Nunez-Smith, M., Wolf, E., Mikiko, Huang, H., Chen, P., Lee, L., Emanuel, E. J., Gross,

C. P. *Media and Child and Adolescent Health: A Systematic Review.* Available online at http://www.commonsensemedia.org/sites/default/files/NunezSmith%20CSM%20media_revi ew%20Dec%204.pdf

Paavonen, E. J., Pennonen, M. & Roine, M. Passive Exposure to TV Linked to Sleep Problems in Children. *Journal of Sleep Research.* 2006; 15: 154-161.

Pagani , L. S., Fitzpatrick, M. A., Barnett, T. A. & Dubow, E. Prospective Associations Between Early Childhood Television Exposure and Academic, Psychosocial, and Physical Well-being by Middle Childhood. *Archives of Pediatric and Adolescent Medicine.* 2010; 164(5): 425-431.

Parush, S., Sohmer, H., Steinberg, A. & Kaitz, M. Somatosensory function in boys with ADHD and tactile defensiveness. *Physiology & Behavior.* 2007;90; 553–558.

Pelligrini, A. D.& Bohn, C. M. The role of recess in children's cognitive performance and school adjustment. *Educational Researcher.* 2005; 34(1): 13-19.

PENT Forum (2008). Available at: http://www.pent.ca.gov/beh/rst/restraintresources.pdf

Petersen, M. C., Kube, D. A. & Palmer, F. B. High prevalence of children with developmental disabilities admitted to a general pediatric inpatient unit. *Journal of Developmental and Physical Disabilities.* 2006; 18 (3): 307-318.

Phillips, C. Medicine Goes to School: Teachers as Sickness Brokers for ADHD. *Public Library of Science Medicine.* 2006; 3(4): e182. Available at: http://www.plosmedicine.org/article/info:doi/10.1371/journal.pmed.0030182

Play TM News. June 5, 2005. *Chinese suicide shows addiction dangers – online life proves too appealing.* By Luke Guttridge. Available at: http://play.tm/news/5928/chinese-suicide-shows-addiction-dangers/

Primack, B. A., Swanier, B., Georgiopoulos, A. M., Land, S. R.& Fine, M. J. Association Between Media Use in Adolescence and Depression in Young Adulthood. *Archives of General Psychiatry.* 2009; 66(2):181-188.

Psychiatric Times. June 26, 2009. By Allen Francis. *A Warning Sign On the Road to the DSMV: Beware of its Unintended Consequences.* Available from: http://www.psychiatrictimes.com/dsm-5/content/article/10168/1425378

Raine ADHD Study: Government of Western Australia - Department of Health. *Long-term outcomes associated with stimulant medication in the treatment of ADHD in children.* http://www.health.wa.gov.au/publications/documents/MICADHD_Raine_ADHD_Study_re port_022010.pdf.

Rapport, M. D., Bolden, J., Kofler, M. J., Sarver, D. E., Raiker, J. S., Alderson, R. M. Hyperactivity in Boys with Attention-Deficit/Hyperactivity Disorder (ADHD): A Ubiquitous Core Symptom or Manifestation of Working Memory Deficits? *Journal of Abnormal Child Psychology.* 2008; DOI 10.1007/s10802-008-9287-8.

Ratey, J. J. & Hagerman, E. *Spark: The Revolutionary New Science of Exercise and the Brain.* Little, Brown and Company, New York. 2008.

Rehbein, F., Kleimann, M. & Mobie, T. Prevalence and Risk Factors of Video Game Dependency in Adolescence: Results of a German Nationwide Study. *Cyberpsychology, Behavior and Social Networking.* 2010;13(3): 269-277. DOI: 10.1089/cyber.2009.0227

Reilly, J. J., Jackson, D. M., Montgomery, C., Kelly, L. A., Slater, C., Grant, S., Paton, J. Y. Total Energy Expenditure and Physical Activity in Young Scottish Children: Mixed Longitudinal Study. *Lancet.* 2004; 363:211-212.

Rideout, V. J., Vandewater, E. A, Wartella, E. A. *Zero to six: electronic media in the lives of infants, toddlers and preschoolers.* Menlo Park (CA): Kaiser Family Foundation; Fall 2003.

Rine, R. M., Braswell, J., Fisher, D., Joyce, K., Kalar, K., Shaffer, M. Improvement of motor development and postural control following intervention in children with sensorineural hearing loss and vestibular impairment. *International Journal of Pediatric Otorhinolaryngology.* 2004; 68, 1141-1148.

Roberts, D.F., Foehr, U. G,, Rideout, V. J., Brodie, M. *Kids and media @ the millennium: A comprehensive national analysis of children's media use.* Menlo Park (CA): Kaiser Family Foundation; 1999.

Robinson, J. P., Martin, S. What Do Happy People Do? *Journal of Social Indicators Research.* 2008; 89:565-571.

Robinson, T. Reducing children's television viewing to prevent obesity. *JAMA.* 1999; 282 (16): 1561-1567.

Rosack, J. Prescription data on youth raise important questions. *American Psychiatric Foundation – Clinical and Research News.* 2003; 38 (3): 1-3.

Rowan, C. Unplug – Don't Drug: A Critical Look at the Influence of Technology on Child Behavior With an Alternative Way of responding Other Than Evaluation and Drugging. *Ethical Human Psychology and Psychiatry.* 2010;12 (1): 60-67.

Ruff,, M. E. Attention Deficit Disorder and stimulant use: An epidemic of modernity. *Clinical Pediatrics.* 2005; 44 (7): 557-563.

Sax, L, & Kauta, K. Who First Suggests the Diagnosis of Attention-Deficit/Hyperactivity Disorder? *Annals of Family Medicine.* 2003; 1(3):171-174. Available at: http://www.annfammed.org/cgi/reprint/1/3/171.

Schaaf, R. D. & Nightlinger, K. M. Occupational therapy using a sensory integrative approach: A case study of effectiveness. *American Journal of Occupational Therapy.* 2007; 61 (2): 239-246.

Shanahan, T. (2007). Early literacy development: Sequence of acquisition. *Encyclopedia of Language and Literacy Development* (pp. 1-6). London, ON: Canadian Language and Literacy Research Network. Retrieved [insert date] from http://www.literacyencyclopedia.ca/pdfs/topic.php?topId=225.

Shao-I, C., Jie-Zhi, L., Der-Hsiang, H. Video Game Addiction in Children and Teenagers in Taiwan. *CyberPsychology and Behavior.* 2004; 7(5):571-581.

Singh, R., Bhalla, A., Lehl, S. S., Sachdev, A. Video game epilepsy. *Neurology India.* 2001;

49 (4): 411-412.

Sloat, E., Willms, J. D. *The International Adult Literacy Survey: Implications for Canadian Social Policy.* Canadian Journal of Education. 2000; 25(3):218-233. Available at: http://www.csse.ca/CJE/Articles/FullText/CJE25-3/CJE25-3-sloat.pdf.

Small, G & Vorgan G. *iBrain: Surviving the technological alternating the modern mind.* Harper Collins Publishers, NY. 2008.

Statistics Canada. 2010. Fitness of Canadian Children and Youth: Results from the 2007-2009 Canadian Health Measures Survey. Retrieved on April 30, 2010 from http://www.statcan.gc.ca/pub/82-003-x/2010001/article/11065/key-cle-eng.htm.

Strauss, R. S. & Pollack, H.A. Epidemic increase in childhood overweight, 1986-1998. *JAMA.* 2001; 286 (22) 2845-2848.

Swanson, J. M., Elliot, G. R., Greenhill, L. L., Wigal, T., Arnold, L. E. & Vitiello, M., Hechtman, L., Epstein, J. N., Pelham, W. E., Abikoff, . B., Newcorn, J., H., Molina, B. S. G., Hinshaw, S., G., Wells, K., C., Hoza, B., Jensen, P. S., Gibbons, R. D., Hur, K., Stehli, A., Davies, M., Marsh, J. S., Connors, C., K., Caron, M. & Volkow, N. D. Effects of Stimulant Medication on Growth Rates Across 3 Years in the MTA Follow-up. *Child and Adolescent Psychiatry.* 2007;46(8);1015-1027. doi:10.1097/chi.0b013e3130686d7e

Swing, E. L., Gentile, D. A., Anderson, C. A. & Walsh, D. A. (2010). Television and Video Game Exposure and the Development of Attention Problems. *Pediatrics.* 126: 214-221. doi: 10.1542/peds.2009-1508

Tannock, M. T. Rough and tumble play: an investigation of the perceptions of educators and young children. *Journal of Early Childhood Education.* 2008; 35: 357-361.

Telegraph, UK. March 5, 2010. *Korean couple let baby starve to death while caring for virtual child.* Available at: http://www.telegraph.co.uk/news/worldnews/asia/southkorea/7376178/Korean-couple-let-baby-starve-to-death-while-caring-for-virtual-child.html

Thomas, C. P., Conrad, P., Casler, R., Goodman, E. Trends in the use of psychotropic medications among adolescents, 1994 to 2001. *Psychiatric Services.* 2006; 57 (1): 63-69.

Tomblin, B. Literacy as an Outcome of Language Development and its Impact on Children's Psychosocial and Emotional Development. *Canadian Language and Literacy Research Network.* 2006. Available at: http://www.literacyencyclopedia.ca.

Tomchek, S. D. & Dunn, W. Sensory Processing in Children With and Without Autism: A Comparative Study Using the Short Sensory Profile. *American Journal of Occupational Therapy.* 61 (2), 190-200.

Tremblay, M. S., Katzmarzyk, P. T., Willms, J. D. Temporal trends in overweight and obesity in Canada, 1981-1996. *International Journal of Obesity.* 2002; 26(4): 538-543.

Tremblay, M. S., Willms, J. D. Is the Canadian childhood obesity epidemic related to physical inactivity? *International Journal of Obesity.* 2005; 27: 1100-1105.

Tronick, E. Neurobehavioral Social Emotional Development in Infants. W. W. Norton &

Co.; UK. 2007.

Turcotte, Martin. *Time spent with family during a typical workday 1986 to 2005*. Statistics Canada. Catalogue No. 11-008. Available from: http://www.statcan.ca/english/freepub/11-008-XIE/2006007/pdf/11-008-XIE20060079574.pdf

United Kingdom Literacy Association. *Reading On Screen*. 2007.

US Consumer Product Safety Commission. Handbook for Public Playground Safety. Washington, DC. http://www.cpsc.gov/cpscpub/pubs/325.pdf.

US Consumer Product Safety Commission. Public Playground Safety Checklist. Washington, DC. http://www.cpsc.gov/cpscpub/pubs/327.html.

Vancouver Sun by Kim Pemberton March 29, 2010. *Violence against school staff is on the rise: Injuries mount as teachers, principals and support workers become targets for assault by students.* Kim Pemberton. Retrieved on August 10, 2010 from http://www.vancouversun.com/news/Violence+against+school+staff+rise/2733827/story.html

Vandewater, E. A., Bickham, D. S., Lee, J. H., Cummings, H. M., Wartella, E. A. & Rideout, V. J. When the television is always on: Heavy television exposure and young children's development. *American Behavioral Scientist*, 2005;48, 562-577.

Vandewater, E. A., Lee, J. H., & Shim, M. Family conflict and violent electronic media use among school-aged children. *Media Psychology*. 2005;7, 73-86.

Viner, R. M., Roche, E., Maguire, S. A. & Nicholls, D. E. Childhood protection and obesity: framework for practice. *British Medical Journal*. 2010;341:c3074; doi:10.1136/bmj.c3074

Vitiello, B. & Towbin, K. Stimulant Treatment of ADHD and Risk of Sudden Death in Children. *Journal of American Psychiatry*. 2009;166; 955-957. doi: 10.1176/appi.ajp.2009.09050619

Waddell C, Hua JM, Garland O, DeV. Peters R, McEwan K. Preventing Mental Disorders in Children: A Systematic Review to Inform Policy-Making. *Canadian Journal of Public Health*. 2007; 98(3): 166-173.

Waddell C. *Improving the Mental Health of Young Children*. Children's Health Policy Centre, Simon Fraser University, Vancouver BC, Canada. 2007. Available at: http://www.firstcallbc.org/pdfs/Communities/4-alliance.pdf.

Waldman, M. *Does Television Cause Autism?* Cornell University. December 2006. Retrieved on April 30, 2010 from http://www.johnson.cornell.edu/faculty/profiles/waldman/autism-waldman-nicholson-adilov.pdf.

Ward S. *Baby Talk*. Arrow Books Ltd, Random House Publishers Group; London, UK. 2004.

Washington Post by Anthony Faiola May 27, 2006. *When Escape Seems Just a Mouse Click Away*. Available at: http://www.washingtonpost.com/wpdyn/content/article/2006/05/26/AR2006052601960.html

Welch, M. G., Northrup, R. S., Welch-Horan, T. B., Ludwig, R. J., Austin, C. L., Jacobson, J. S. Outcomes of prolonged parent-child embrace therapy among 102 children with behavior disorders. *Complementary Therapies in Clinical Practice.* 2006; 12(1): 3-12.

Willard N. E. The Authority and Responsibility of School Officials in Responding to *Cyberbullying. Journal of Adolescent Health.* 2007; 41:S64-65.

Willms, J. D. *Vulnerable Children.* University of Alberta Press; Edmonton. 2002.

Winterstein, A. G., Gerhard, T., Shuster, J., Saidi,A. Cardiac Safety of Methylphenidate Versus Amphetamine Salts in the Treatment of ADHD. *Pediatrics.* 2009; 124 (1): e75-e80.

Worthen, M.R. Education Policy Implications from the Expert Panel on Electronic Media and Youth Violence. *Journal of Adolescent Health.* 2007; 41:S61-63.

Xiuquin, H., Huimin, Z., Mengchen, L., Jinan, W., Ying, Z. and Ran, T. Mental Health, Personality, and Parental Rearing Styles of Adolescents with Internet Addiction Disorder. *Cyberpsychology, Behavior, and Social Networking.* 2010. DOI: 10.1089/cyber.2009.0222

Ybarra, M. L., Diener-West, M., Leaf, P. J. Examining the Overlap in Internet Harassment and School Bullying: Implications for School Intervention. *Journal of Adolescent Health.* 2007; 41:S42-S50.

Yen, J. Y., Yen, C. F., Chen, C. S., Tang T. C., Ko, C. H. The Association between Adult ADHD Symptoms and Internet Addiction among College Students: The Gender Difference. *CyberPsychology & Behavior.* 2008: doi:10.1089/cpb.2008.0113.

Zimmerman, F. J., Christakis, D. A., Meltzoff, A. N. Television and DVD/video viewing in children younger than 2 years. *Archives of Pediatric Adolescent Medicine.* 2007; 161 (5): 473-479.

Zito, J. M., Safer, D. J., dosReis, S., Gardner, J. F., Boles, M., Lynch, F. Trends in the prescribing of psychotropic medications to preschoolers. *JAMA.* 2000; 283: 1025-1030.

Zito, J. M., Safer, D. J., dosReis, S., Gardner, J. F., Soeken, K., Boles, M., Lynch, F. Rising prevalence of antidepressants among US youth. *Pediatrics.* 2002; 109 (5): 721-727.

Zito, J. M., Safer, D. J, dosReis S., Gardner, J. F., Magder, L., Soeken , K., Lynch, F, Riddle, M. Psychotropic practice patterns for youth. *Archives of Pediatric and Adolescent Medicine.* 2003; 157(1): 17-25.

Index

Acknowledgements

First and foremost, I would like to thank the children, parents, teachers, and therapists who so graciously shared their most intimate thoughts and ideas regarding technology and its impact on children. Secondly, I would like to thank my exquisite editorial staff which consisted of my husband and editor in chief Ian, son and wise mentor Matt, mom and counselor extraordinaire Val, guide and muse Cheryl, astute thinker and healer Jody, kayak and nature buddy Tracy, and nephew and future lawyer Nick. Although she was not on my editorial staff, I would like to thank my daughter Katie who painstakingly did all the graphics for all of my programs, and suffered through many long and arduous discussions about technology and children. Without all of you, this book would have been possible, but would have taken me a lot longer to perfect! Thank you!

Author Biography

Cris Rowan is an impassioned pediatric occupational therapist who has first-hand understanding and knowledge of how technology can cause profound changes in a child's development, behavior and their ability to learn. An activist for change and frequent guest on CBC radio, and featured on CBC TV's *Doc Zone* documentary called *Are We Digital Dummies* on November 18, 2010, Cris has broadcast her plans for a "balanced" future to millions.

Cris has Bachelor of Science degrees in both Occupational Therapy and Biology, and is a SIPT certified sensory integration specialist. Cris is a member in good standing with the BC College of Occupational Therapists, and has over 20 years experience working with children in home, school and clinic based settings.

CEO of *Sunshine Coast Occupational Therapy Inc.* and *Zone'in Programs Inc.*, Cris offers products, workshops, training and consultation services to improve child health and enhance academic performance. Cris designed *Zone'in, Move'in, Unplug'in* and *Live'in* educational products for elementary children to address the rise in developmental delays, and behavior disorders from technology overuse. Cris has performed over 200 *Foundation Series Workshops* on topics such as sensory integration and attention, motor development and literacy, attachment formation and addictions, early intervention, technology overuse, media literacy programs, and school environmental design for the 21st century for teachers, parents and health professionals throughout North America.

Cris has recently created *Zone'in Training Programs* to train other pediatric occupational therapists to deliver these integral workshops in their own community. Cris is an expert reviewer for the Canadian Family Physician Journal, authors the monthly *Zone'in Development Series Newsletter* and is author of the following initiatives: *Unplug – Don't Drug, Creating Sustainable Futures Program*, and *Linking Corporations to Community*.

Cris is the proud parent of two lovely children, and lives in the beautiful and remote village of Sechelt in British Columbia, Canada, with her husband, daughter, 2 dogs, 3 cats, parrot and horse.

CPSIA information can be obtained at www.ICGtesting.com
Printed in the USA
LVOW05s1143221013

358035LV00005B/110/P